CW01496872

FALSE CURE

FALSE CURE

The Miracle Cream Fueling
a Denied Epidemic—and the
Movement Fighting Back

KELLY PALACE
M.ED., ITSAN CO-FOUNDER

Copyright © 2025 by Kelly Palace

All rights reserved. No part of this book may be reproduced, distributed, or transmitted in any form or by any means—electronic, mechanical, photocopying, recording, or otherwise—without prior written permission of the author. For permissions: **www.KellyPalace.com**

First Edition, 2025

ISBN: 979-8-9930947-0-0

Front cover design by Tom Drysdale
Back cover and interior design by SHR Book Design

This book is a work of nonfiction. Some names and identifying details have been changed to protect privacy.

Medical Disclaimer: This book is not intended to provide medical advice, diagnosis, or treatment. It is for informational and educational purposes only. Readers should not rely on the information in this book as a substitute for professional medical advice, diagnosis, or treatment.

Artificial Intelligence (AI) Assistance Disclaimer: AI tools were used to support grammar, punctuation, research, and style in *False Cure*. The experiences, narratives, ideas, and source confirmations are entirely the author's. The author takes full responsibility for the book's content and accuracy. The cover art and formatting were produced by human designers who also used AI responsibly, with no copyright violations.

To **Dr. Marvin J. Rapaport**:
physician, pioneer, and the whistleblower
for the thousands whose suffering was
dismissed, misdiagnosed, or denied.

This book—and the movement it represents—would
not exist without your life's work that lit the path for
us and gave us answers, strength, and healing.

And **to those in the throes of healing**, *and to*
those who have endured this crisis—you are the
reason this injustice must be exposed.
Your suffering is not in vain.

CONTENTS

Part V ✦ The Resistance

Part VI ✦ The Advocates and Activists

PREFACE

THIS BOOK IS BORN OUT OF A CONVERGENCE of experiences few could claim. My family has many medical doctors. I spent a decade inside Pfizer Pharmaceuticals, the world's largest drug company, writing for its internal magazine and calling on physicians as part of its sales force. I became a patient of the pioneering whistleblowing doctor who first identified topical steroid addiction and withdrawal. I have lived through this condition myself and studied it for two decades. I am a journalist, an author, and co-founder of the International Topical Steroid Awareness Network (ITSAN). These experiences together give me a perspective no one else could bring to this story.

The truth cannot be told without naming the medical establishment itself as at fault. Each time journalists, news outlets, the FDA, eczema associations, or young doctors have "looked into" topical steroid withdrawal, they went to the same source for answers: dermatologists. And for decades, the answer was the same—*"This condition does not exist."* More recently: *"It's rare"* or *"just a worsening rash."*

That refrain has kept an epidemic hidden—actually denied. Topical steroid addiction is an iatrogenic condition: caused not by disease, but by the treatment itself. And the truth is painfully simple—the very doctors who caused the harm have been the least willing, and often the least able, to admit it. To do so would be to admit responsibility.

Some doctors in these pages are quoted in ways that show them as dismissive, evasive, or even willfully misleading. But I want to be clear: I carry a deep respect for medicine. My family's "wall of doctors" displays photos of five generations of physicians—my great-grand-father, grandfather, father's siblings, my brother, a niece and nephew. Medicine has always been revered in my family.

This book is not anti-medicine. I trust and use medicine—I completed my COVID vaccinations, receive my annual flu shot, and I was treated for breast cancer. This book is anti-denial, anti-gaslighting, and anti-harm when treatments are pushed past their safe limits.

Another reason I must write this book: I became a patient. Not just anyone's patient, but one of Dr. Marvin J. Rapaport—the first dermatologist to expose topical steroid withdrawal. My own journey was devastating. For years, my skin burned, peeled, oozed, and itched until daily life was unbearable. The suffering was unlike anything "eczema" could explain. But I healed. Today my skin is healthier than ever—living proof of recovery. My experience is replicated by millions worldwide. When these powerful hormone-based drugs are stopped, healing begins—though only after a harrowing crisis.

My exposure didn't stop there. In 2009, I launched *AddictedSkin.org*, one of the first lifelines for patients searching for answers, alongside Dr. Rapaport and his research. In 2012 we co-founded ITSAN. I served as its first president, uniting patients globally and pushing a silenced epidemic into the light. I have lived in the trenches of this condition—first as a patient, then as a leader, now as a witness for millions.

PREFACE

This book is not written in anger, though anger would be justified. It is guided by investigation—to prove that this condition is not rare, but epidemic. **I welcome scrutiny: every claim is sourced, every quote is traceable, and where the record is anecdotal, I'll tell you and you can be the judge.** I will present clinical studies, case histories, and the stories of families broken. This is not activism. It is journalism.

You'll also hear from the few courageous dermatologists and general practitioners who dared to stand with patients—proof that medicine can course-correct when truth is allowed in. My journalism degree trained me to investigate; my years with Pfizer taught me how the system works; my role with ITSAN revealed the scale of harm. And my own skin—and the suffering I've witnessed, especially among children—made it impossible to look away.

This book is for the patients still suffering, the caregivers standing beside them, the doctors willing to listen, and anyone who has ever trusted a prescription pad. It is for skeptics. I hope doubters will see the patterns, the evidence, the human toll—and then the light.

The chapters ahead are divided into six sections: *The Awakening, The Proof, The Human Toll, The Fight Ignites, The Resistance,* and *The Advocates and Activists*—each tracing a different dimension of this denied epidemic and the movement that rose against it, from denial to resistance, and from patient suffering to advocacy.

Read with an open mind and an open heart. **Because once you see what has been hidden, you cannot unsee it. And you may save someone you love from a *False Cure*.**

INVITATION TO DOCTORS

A message from your patients:
This book is not just history or evidence; it is our invitation to you—from the patients who have lived this suffering and who know that courage can change everything.

TO THOSE WHO TOOK AN OATH TO "*DO NO HARM*":

We know some of you see it—the telltale signs of patients suffering from Topical Steroid Addiction and/or Withdrawal. You hear our stories, you hear about our skin burning, reddening, and rashes spreading. You notice the patterns that don't fit the textbook. And yet, speaking out is hard. You feel the eyes of your peers and the weight of your profession pressing you to look away. Naming this for what it is can feel risky. Medical dogma is real.

But you are not alone. Around the world, more and more doctors are breaking the silence. Many of the doctors in this book broke that silence decades ago. We hope you'll read the history of how we got here, and what is happening around the world. Many doctors have already stood where you are standing now, facing the same doubts and fears—and they chose to act.

We ask you to trust what you already know in your heart. Follow your instincts. You know something is terribly wrong. Find the courage to call it by its name. Guide your patients where little guidance exists. Stand on the right side of history. Your oath matters. Your voice matters. Your patients need you.

What Changed My Mind

"Patients often come in telling us that they have TSW, and that is a big reversal for dermatology. We're not built for that, and it can feel threatening. But I've come to see it differently. Listening to patients and observing the different patterns in their skin has changed my mind. I love those moments in life when my mind gets changed—it's very exciting."

—Peter A. Lio, MD, Clinical Assistant Professor of Dermatology and Pediatrics, Northwestern University Feinberg School of Medicine

INTRODUCTION

||||||||||||||||||||||||||||||||||||||||||||||||||||||||||||||||||||||||||||||||||||||||||||||||||||||||||||||||||||||||||||||||||

WHAT IF THE COMMON SKIN CREAM IN YOUR medicine cabinet is destroying your health?

What if your doctor prescribes you an even stronger one, without the warnings it should carry?

Topical steroids are everywhere. Hydrocortisone, Cortaid, prescriptions for eczema or psoriasis. They're sold over the counter, handed out casually by doctors like candy, and hidden in cosmetic products like makeup, skin lighteners, and fade creams. They're used on bug bites, rashes, acne, poison ivy—even on babies—without a second thought.

But these drugs have triggered one of the most devastating and ignored health crises of our time, affecting **every age and every color of skin**. An estimated **3.8 million Americans**—and countless more worldwide—are suffering from **Topical Steroid Addiction and Withdrawal (TSA/TSW)**.

False Cure is the whistleblowing story of that crisis, and the movement that rose, and is still rising, to expose it.

FALSE CURE

You may think this is just a book about skin. It isn't. Steroids run quietly through nearly every corner of modern medicine: an inhaler, an eyedrop, a nasal spray, a cortisone shot in a painful shoulder or knee, a cream in the bathroom drawer. Each one seems harmless, but the body keeps score. Steroid exposure is cumulative, invisible, and often unchecked. What begins as a cream for a rash can end as a lifetime of hidden harm. *False Cure* exposes not just a skin crisis, but a systemic one—and no family is untouched.

This book pulls back the curtain on how a "miracle cream" ignited a global health nightmare. You'll see how regulators, doctors, and the organizations meant to protect us—the National Eczema Association, the American Academy of Dermatology, the FDA—looked the other way, ignoring both patients and published science. You'll meet the few courageous doctors who defied the system to tell the truth. And you'll meet the influencers and survivors whose pain turned into a global call for justice.

The topical steroid market was valued at $5.2 billion in 2024 and is expected to grow to $7.2 billion by 2033 (Verified Market Research). And that doesn't include the hidden black-market creams flooding stores and online. The problem isn't shrinking; it's expanding.

This book is for every parent, patient, and practitioner who has ever been told: *"It's just eczema." "This cream is safe."*

It's not.

The truth? TSA/TSW recovery can take two to five years—or more—of burning, oozing, insomnia, and bone-deep itching. It can bring isolation, despair, and mental health collapse. And yet it is all preventable.

Finally, here is a book that names the problem, documents the harm, and honors the people who refused to stay silent. A book you can hand to a doctor, a friend, or a loved one and say: *This is real. This is happening. And it must end.*

For millions, it begins with an itch. And a miracle cream.

PART I

THE AWAKENING

CHAPTER ONE

IT STARTED WITH AN ITCH

||||||||||||||||||||||||||||||||||||||||||||||||||||||||||||||||||||||||||||||||||||||||||||||||||||||||||||||||||||||||||||||||||||||||

WHEN I WAS A LITTLE GIRL, I wore my swimsuit to bed because my mom couldn't get me out of it, so she just let me sleep in it.

I loved being in my bathing suit and loved the idea of being a swimmer. It was like the kids you see wearing their Superman costumes in the grocery store.

My swimsuit was (and still is) my superhero costume. I want to always be ready to swim.

I adore everything about swimming. The lights reflecting off the surface of the water. The sound of my breath blowing bubbles. Being beneath the surface in a quiet world of its own. I feel most at home in the water.

At the young age that I wore my swimsuit to bed, I didn't yet go to early morning swim practices. But it was that same burning passion and newly acquired skills that carried me forward—drive, discipline, joy—all of it led me to become the kind of teenager who would wake up at 4:15 a.m. for morning workouts. I was striving to be like the Olympic heroes I watched on television. It was Shane

Gould of Australia, Shirley Babashoff of the U.S., and of course Mark Spitz, who particularly inspired me. That's when I set my mind to train for the Olympics. I was 12 years old.

And that's when the itching started.

I noticed it mostly at night—a small, slightly bumpy rash between my fingers. Barely visible, but deeply annoying. It didn't affect my swimming, my school, or my social life in any meaningful way. It just itched. And only at night, for some reason. I couldn't have it keeping me awake when I needed my precious sleep for a hard morning swim practice.

One of my fellow swimmers' father was a well-known dermatologist in our area—Dr. "L", as we called him. When I visited his office with my mom, he wasn't concerned about my rash at all. He said I had eczema. Eczema is a common skin condition which today affects 31 million Americans. There are several different types of eczema, two common types are, atopic dermatitis, a chronic, genetic condition linked to immune dysfunction, and contact dermatitis, a temporary skin reaction caused by direct exposure to an irritant or allergen.

Anyone can get contact dermatitis—it's not genetic, and it can happen to otherwise healthy individuals of any age. Without trying to discover which type I might have had, he handed me a prescription for what would be a large tube of cream and confidently said, *"This is a miracle cream. It'll take away your itch."*

It worked like a charm.

And it came with unlimited refills.

The prescription cream was for Diprosone, a mid-to-high potency topical steroid, although we had no idea of this at the time. He assured us it was *"safe enough to put on a baby."*

So I kept the tube on my nightstand. When I'd wake up scratching in the middle of the night, I'd roll over, half-asleep, dab it on my fingers, and drift off again before my alarm could wake me.

This was 1973.

Sadly and disturbingly, not much has changed in how dermatologists treat eczema today, over 50 years later.

1979 was a significant year for me as it was my high school graduation year, but it was also very important as a landmark clinical paper on the dangers of topical steroids was published. We'll get there in a minute.

For the next four years of high school, I lived in a swirl of chlorine, anxiety, and trying to fit in. I was that girl who seemed to have it together on the outside—varsity swimmer, lifeguard in the summers, ran track, even was a cheerleader. But under the surface, I was paddling hard. I was bullied more than most people knew. Anxiety and panic disorder often followed me through the halls like shadows I couldn't shake. Still, I kept showing up—at practice, at meets, at school—and somehow kept believing that better days were ahead. When I graduated, I was ready for a fresh start. College swimming and a journalism degree felt like more than just the next step—they felt like freedom.

And all that time in the chlorine paid off, because in the summer before I headed off to college, I set one of my first notable records—a U.S. Swimming National Distance Record in the 4-mile Cable-Swim at Chris Greene Lake in Virginia—a bright achievement in what felt like a time of promise and possibility. Many friends from my club team swam that race with me and we celebrated until after midnight that night.

In my not-so-distant future there would be another past-midnight moment that had a much darker theme. You'll hear about that later in this chapter.

A Young Journalist

Sometimes people ask me how I remember historic moments from my past, like the ones I'm recounting here, or in my previous book. The answer is simple: I've always been a prolific journal writer. Every night, I sit down to record the significant events of my day—often detailing the nuances of each lap I swam during practice, what my workday included, or something entertaining my friends or family did.

I had no idea at the time that these seemingly ordinary moments, captured in ink on paper back then—or on my phone now—would one day weave themselves into the tapestry of my career as a story-teller, carrying with them echoes of lessons and messages to share far beyond my own experience.

And just like journaling was a nightly routine back then, through high school I continued to get refills of the "miracle cream." I'd rub it on my hands at night, just like always, whenever the itching came back. It was so normalized, so trusted, it felt like brushing my teeth. This practice was doctor-prescribed and approved.

Little did I know, this was the beginning of an addiction. But not the kind you might think.

Now that landmark clinical paper I mentioned. 1979 was the year dermatology quietly issued one of its earliest warnings about topical steroids.

That year, researchers Kligman and Frosch published a ground-breaking paper titled *Steroid Addiction* in the *Archives of Dermatology*, Volume 115, Issue 4, April 1979, describing what they called an "in-sidious type of side reaction" linked to long-term use of topical ste-roids. They documented how patients could develop symptoms like persistent redness, itching, scaling, and skin thinning—symptoms that often worsened after stopping the creams. They warned that this withdrawal pattern was going unrecognized by both patients and physicians. But neither these researchers nor the American Academy of Dermatology did anything in response. In fact, they did the opposite of what would have benefited patients. They ramped up steroid usage for all inflammatory conditions.

It was, essentially, an early medical recognition of what is known as Red Skin Syndrome, or Topical Steroid Addiction and Topical Steroid Withdrawal Syndrome. All three of these are used interchangeably to describe this horrible condition that occurs when one's skin becomes addicted to steroids. In this book, I'll refer to topical steroid addiction as TSA and topical steroid withdrawal as TSW.

And just to clarify, when I say "steroids" throughout, I'm referring to corticosteroids—not anabolic steroids. Those are the kind that make bodybuilders look like action figures. My apologies for the medical jargon, but don't worry—there won't be any heavy charts or graphs to put you to sleep. In fact, you won't find a single picture in this book, because let's face it, the internet is already brimming with incredible photos and videos on this subject. This book is all about people and policies, and whistleblowing. So trust me, coming up are some real-life encounters with professional medical personnel and organizational regulatory leaders that will have you shaking your head. This is a case of truth being stranger than fiction.

Back to Dr. Kligman—a great researcher—but he didn't pay it forward. Though celebrated for his dermatologic discoveries, his career was also marred by controversy over unethical prisoner experiments in the mid-20th century, a shadow that complicates his legacy. But his contributions and discoveries are still considered valuable.

This is a direct quote from Dr. Albert Kligman's clinical paper, *Steroid Addiction*. His description is haunting—and it was written nearly 50 years ago:

> **Addiction to topical steroids is a serious problem, which reaches tragic proportions in some cases.** *It is more common than realized. It slyly seduces, and this will be prevented only when the physician becomes as impressed with the capacity of the steroids to do harm as with their power to suppress inflammation and cure virtually any inflammatory disorder.*

Dr. Kligman's *Steroid Addiction* warning article was simply forgotten. The signs were there. The concerns were raised. But nothing changed. Doctors kept prescribing. Patients kept trusting. And the creams kept coming...

Unfortunately, it was not Dr. Kligman who took up the mantle to prevent the tragedy of Topical Steroid Addiction. That task would fall to another doctor in Chapter 3.

CHAPTER TWO

DOWN THE RABBIT HOLE

AS YOU READ THIS NEXT STORY, KNOW THAT there are millions of people across the country—and around the world—going through the exact same thing I'm about to describe. They are going through it right now. Lost. Alone. Suffering.

My story is not unique. I know this now after deeply studying and experiencing the topic for over 20 years. **Being gaslit, dismissed, and made sicker by a failing medical system is sadly not rare.** My experience shows what happened to a health-conscious, educated adult in excellent health. But what about the children? The elderly? The exhausted parents just trying to help their loved ones?

For most of my years in my 20s and 30s, I still had mild rashes on my hands and, on rare occasions, around my eyes and mouth. I always treated these with either over-the-counter topical steroid creams—like the hydrocortisone you can buy at the drugstore—or with something prescribed by a dermatologist. Either kept my skin in check.

Then, in my early forties, I had one of those random, run-of-the-mill flare-ups around my eyes—probably from a new pair of swim goggles that I tightened too much and the plastic didn't agree with my sensitive eyelids. Just a little red and itchy. Nothing major.

It's possible that what I had around my eyes was only contact dermatitis, which goes away on its own. A simple skin reaction to a new pair of goggles. The truth is, anyone can get contact dermatitis. It's not genetic. It's not chronic. It's not some mysterious autoimmune puzzle. It's a reaction—your skin saying "no thank you" to a soap, a fabric, a chemical, or yes, a pair of overly tight swim goggles.

And here's the thing: contact dermatitis usually clears on its own in under two weeks, without any medication at all. No steroid required.

Which means a rash like this wasn't just a rash—it could be a trap–for anyone. Because even a healthy person with no history of the atopic dermatitis kind of eczema can walk into a doctor's office with a little redness... and walk out with a powerful topical steroid. That's how easy it is to become a casualty—not of eczema itself, but of the treatment. When you're not careful—or not informed—you don't just treat a rash. You risk starting a cycle that's hard to stop. A slippery slope disguised as a solution. A false cure.

If Only I Had a Time Machine

During a routine eye exam, my doctor tilted her head, squinted, and said, "Want me to prescribe something that will clear up that rash around your eyes?"

I said yes before she even finished the sentence. She never mentioned it was a steroid. I didn't ask. Two days later, my eyelids were smooth as a dolphin. Another miracle cream, I thought.

Armed with unlimited refills, I dabbed it on whenever I felt a little dryness. It was easy, effective, even luxurious—like a fancy French moisturizer that happened to erase rashes.

But within weeks, the rash crept to my hairline, upper lip, chin. My eyes crusted and swelled. Every time I tried to stop, I flared. A flare is an exacerbation of symptoms, in case you didn't know that. It was getting old putting ice on my eyes to get the swelling down every morning, so I headed off to the dermatologist.

Just a note here. Do you ever play the game, if I could go back in time and change something in my life? Well, this would be the moment. Remember, all I had was a great life and a little rash on my eyelids before my spiral into hell was caused by doctors who believe that topical steroids are safe enough to put on a baby!

The hellish condition I was about to descend into is called Topical Steroid Addiction and it's an Iatrogenic condition. I know I promised, no boring science, but this is a cool word you may want to remember for your next scrabble game, iatrogenic means a condition caused by a medical treatment. Mine's a typical path for millions, all 100 percent approved by the American Academy of Dermatology.

Dermatologist #1: The Shot Giver

I saw my first dermatologist. Let's call her The Shot Giver. She injected me with a Kenolog shot (prednisone) and also gave me more steroid creams. My skin cleared up for a few weeks—until it didn't. The flares returned, more intense than before and spreading to more parts of my body.

Dermatologist #2: The Dismissive

Next up, The Dismissive. She said my skin looked like an infection (it wasn't) and told me to keep using the steroid cream. No questions, no concern about duration or potency. But a nice course of antibiotics, which gave me a yeast infection and diarrhea. My skin kept getting worse.

Dermatologist #3: The Big-City Hope

In desperation, I drove to Orlando to see a highly recommended dermatologist—The Big-City Hope. This time I thought I'd be able to find the right doctor. But the doctor was not lucky for me. Friends had watched my health deteriorate and begged me to try him. But he brushed aside how much steroid I'd already used and prescribed something stronger. He gave me something for my entire face, called it "mild." Safe. Daily use approved. The same messaging drilled into him at med school.

Despite my instincts, I followed his orders. I smeared the cream across my entire face. I tried to wean off. But the moment I stopped? Red, swollen, burning skin. I was stuck in a cyclical hell—a living nightmare of flares, fear, and dependency. Desperate. I tried yet another doctor.

Dermatologist #4: The Parasite Prophet

Enter The Parasite Prophet. She diagnosed—wait for it—scabies.

Yes. Scabies. Something more likely caught in a prison than the local swimming pool.

She prescribed Permethrin, a thick, toxic-smelling cream.

Directions? "Cover your entire body and sleep in it overnight." My husband was required to be treated as well, even though he didn't have so much as a hangnail. We boiled sheets, scrubbed doorknobs, treated our home like a CDC hot zone.

And of course... it didn't help. It burned. It reeked. And the label? "May cause nerve damage."

From a cream I didn't need. For a parasite I didn't have. If I hadn't been in so much pain, I would've screamed. Instead, I cried, stared at the ceiling and side-eyed my husband like we were in a zombie apocalypse.

That night, we were coated in goo, stinky and miserable. My husband looked at me, half-laughing, half-heartbroken, and said, "I think we've reached a new low point."

We hadn't. I think the toxic scabies cream further damaged my already sensitive skin over my whole body because now I was red and raw everywhere. I had to find a doctor that could help me.

Dermatologist #5: The Tub of Doom

Soon after, I saw Dr. Tub of Doom. This one prescribed the full-body "soak and smear" using Triamcinolone—a mid strength topical steroid ointment that comes in a 1-pound jar.

I got a prescription for SIX one-pound jars.

Yes. You read that right: six pounds of steroids! Let that sink in. A mid-strength topical steroid is distributed in one-pound jars. This wasn't medicine. There is nothing judicious about that. It was madness.

My husband helped apply it, wearing latex gloves like we were in a biohazard scene. I used it three times. Each time, the rash and redness would disappear for a few days to weeks, but return worse than before.

This was in 2009, but the practice hasn't changed. As recently as the spring of 2025, I heard a dermatologist on a podcast recall that during his training he was told: "Triamcinolone is your BEST friend—and it comes in a one-pound jar." That's a direct quote.

Nothing was working. I was exhausted. Suicidal thoughts crept in. I no longer cared if I lived or died.

My Mental Health Unraveled

I had once been an avid triathlete. But now? Movement triggered flares. I became housebound. Isolated. My skin burned from head to toe.

Still, I kept searching. I saw 20+ providers: allergists, internists, acupuncturists, energy healers, hypnotists—even a colon hydro-therapist. Yes, I got my rear-end hooked up to a reverse aquatic vacuum and was told I had "trapped trauma" in my bowels.

I remember thinking, *If my skin doesn't kill me, the shame of this moment might. But at least my colon was clean.*

We spent $12,000 out-of-pocket on these specialists. Twelve. Thousand. Dollars. And my face was still on fire.

Labs said I was "healthy as a horse." But my body? Covered in red, burning, weeping skin.

The Rosacea Detour

At some point, I convinced myself it was Rosacea—maybe even steroid-induced. I asked my GP for help. He gave me Metrogel. It cost $120. Burned my skin. Didn't help.

Because I didn't have Rosacea. I had steroid-induced eczema. But no one knew. Not even me.

We tried everything. Elimination diets. Juice fasts. Allergen purges. We even lived with my parents for months to rule out household mold.

I became paranoid. Was it the sun? The air? The drywall?

At one point, I drove wearing a floppy hat, sunglasses, and a damp bandana—like I was robbing a bank. A guy at a stoplight gave me a thumbs-up. I never figured out if it was solidarity or fear.

In just two years leading up to 2009, I was prescribed topical, oral, or injected steroids 14 times.

Cracks in the Cure

Finally, I read an article about corticosteroids causing Cushing's Syndrome and hip necrosis. Teenagers were getting hip replacements.

That hit me hard. I was in my mid-forties worrying about artificial hips. Something was deeply wrong. So I tried to stop the steroids every now and then, but couldn't endure the resulting flares.

Then one of my weeks off steroids my blood pressure plummeted, my GP casually said, "You might be having an adrenal crisis."

Excuse me?

A life-threatening collapse of vital hormones, tossed out like a weather forecast. That was the final straw.

Midnight Searches

This was the late night moment I was in the darkest place yet, so I turned to the internet hoping against hope I could find something.

I had been in pharmaceutical sales for over a decade. I knew how to do research. So I stayed up late digging through journals, articles and studies.

That's when I found it:

"Eyelid Dermatitis to Red Skin Syndrome to Cure" by a Beverly Hills dermatologist named Dr. Marvin Rapaport.

The case studies matched my story. Line for line. Word for word.

At the bottom of the article? The author of the paper's email address.

I took a breath, poured my soul into a cry for help and hit send. It was 12:30 a.m. My fingers trembled. The computer screen glowed in the dark.

Just minutes later, he replied:

"You are not crazy. You are not alone. You can heal."

He must have been on his computer at the same time. With the details I gave him, he diagnosed me via email. Red Skin Syndrome. Told me I had topical steroid addiction—and gave me the one pre-scription no one else had: stop all steroids, for good. No tapering. Stop all steroids. No going back. They are all cumulative. This would turn out to be the real miracle, not the false miracle cream.

That night, I found a lifeline. Who was this man who said I could heal—who understood what was happening to my body when dozens of doctors did not?

CHAPTER THREE

THE DOCTOR WHO DARED

||||||||||||||||||||||||||||||||||||||||||||||||||||||||||||||||||||||||||||||||||||||||||||||||||||||||||||||||||||||||||||||||||||||||||||||||||||||

EVERY REVOLUTION STARTS WITH ONE PERSON who refuses to look away.

It was Sunday, August 17th, 2008. Dr. Marvin Rapaport, a dermatologist located in Beverly Hills, California, urgently picked up the phone in his office and dialed the burn unit of the August Children's Hospital in Philadelphia—he needed to speak directly with one of the attending physicians. But he wasn't having any luck getting through. He had just received an urgent and disturbing email from a frantic father. He knew he was the only doctor who could help this family's tragic situation. So he hopped on a plane from L.A. to N.J. the morning of August 18th, 2008.

A little girl's life was at stake.

Rachel was only eleven years old and weighed just sixty pounds. Her skin was raw, purple, oozing, and covered in open wounds. She had been hospitalized for months, in and out of the ICU, pumped full of painkillers and steroids—oral, topical, and inhaled. Now she was in the burn unit of a Pennsylvania hospital. The doctors didn't know what was wrong with her skin. So they wrapped her in topical steroids. More steroids. More sedatives. More confusion.

Rachel's father, desperate and sleepless, typed three words into Google that changed everything: *Prednisone Withdrawal Symptoms.* The search led him to a name he had never heard before—Dr. Marvin Rapaport.

When Dr. Rapaport saw Rachel's case, he was furious. She wasn't infected or burned. She wasn't crazy. One of the doctors had told her it was all in her head. She was being poisoned by the very medications meant to help her. Her symptoms were textbook Topical Steroid Addiction. But no one at the hospital would listen.

On his own dime, without being asked, Dr. Rapaport flew across the country and walked into the burn unit where Rachel lay. He stood beside her bed—a tiny, lifeless child who once had nothing but mild eczema, now on life support. Her skin was so fragile she couldn't bear the touch of a fingertip. Her parents took turns sleeping at the Ronald McDonald House while fighting every doctor who tried to give her just one more dose of steroids.

She had already been misdiagnosed, misunderstood, and mutilated by medicine.

He was the first one to say: *Stop everything.*

Rapaport had to say it in person because no one believed him otherwise. This was one of the worst cases he had ever seen. It made him angry—not just for Rachel, but for every patient who could end up like her. Rapaport was stunned that a world-renowned institution like the Children's Hospital of Philadelphia could fail to recognize and treat topical steroid addiction.

What she needed wasn't more drugs—it was time, ice, rest, and above all: belief.

Dr. Rapaport told Rachel's parents to hang on. He gave them hope and assurance that their little girl wasn't dying from some strange disease. She was withdrawing from steroids. He made four trips in total from Los Angeles to visit Rachel until she was out of the woods.

And she survived.

I spoke with Rachel after she was fully healed and grown up. She reflected on the five years she spent in and out of hospitals—missing school, enduring isolation, being bullied for how her skin looked, and witnessing traumatic scenes in the burn unit that no child should ever have to see.

"Dr. Rapaport was a knight in shining armor," she told me. "He absolutely saved my life, and I am indebted to him forever."

Her words—simple and true—carry the weight of every child still trapped in the system that nearly cost her everything.

Rachel's story was not an isolated tragedy—it was a preview of what happens when the medical system refuses to see what's right in front of it. And though I didn't know it at the time, I was following a similar path.

In my midnight moment when I closed Dr. Rapaport's email, I felt two things: terror and hope. I didn't know it yet, but Dr. Marvin Rapaport had been fighting this battle for decades.

At a time when nearly every dermatologist in the world was reaching for topical steroids as a standard fix, Dr. Rapaport was quietly noticing something others were ignoring. He saw a pattern: patients who used topical steroids for extended periods were not getting better—they were getting worse. The very medicine prescribed to soothe and heal was, over time, turning the skin against itself.

But no one wanted to hear that.

When I first met Dr. Rapaport in 2009, he was in his seventies—a seasoned dermatologist with the steady gaze of someone who had seen everything. **Yet then—and now, pushing ninety—there is still fire in his voice.** And as of 2025, he is still practicing, still answering calls from desperate patients, still unwilling to set down the burden that most of his peers have ignored.

He often reflects on his early years in medicine and points out something striking: in those days, adult eczema was virtually nonexistent. Children usually grew out of it. What he sees now—today's epidemic of adults trapped in chronic rashes, and children whose eczema only worsens with treatment—he believes is not eczema at all, but the signature of a drug: steroid-induced eczema, or steroid addiction.

In the 1970s, Dr. Rapaport began his career as an assistant clinical professor and researcher at UCLA. There he originated and founded the Allergy, Contact Dermatitis, and Photosensitivity Clinic, where he began seeing patients who didn't fit the mold. They came with classic signs of eczema, but their conditions defied logic and resisted treatment. When he took a detailed history, the common denominator was chronic steroid use. These patients had been diagnosed and re-diagnosed, patched up with stronger prescriptions, injections, and pills. Still, they returned—angrier rashes, angrier skin, and far too often, emotional despair. They were getting worse, not better.

Most doctors dismissed these cases as severe or "recalcitrant" eczema. But Dr. Rapaport looked deeper. He saw what others wouldn't: the steroid creams were no longer helping—they were harming. And he noticed there was a distinct difference between eczema and topical steroid addiction. TSA patients have skin that is more red, often spreading to new parts of the body, and—importantly—the skin has a burning sensation, which is uncharacteristic of eczema. There was also elephant skin, body temperature issues, and excessive shedding of the skin.

He began documenting his findings and, over the years, wrote and published six peer-reviewed papers on the subject of topical steroid addiction, what he came to call Red Skin Syndrome. He named it this because the patients he saw were red. One of his most poignant and practical publications, *Corticosteroid addiction and withdrawal in the atopic: The red burning skin syndrome* (*Clinics in Dermatology*, 2003), laid out not only the trajectory of this iatrogenic condition (one caused by medical treatment), but also a roadmap for healing. His publications became the foundation for Japanese, Indian, and British physicians who documented the same withdrawal syndrome in their own patients.

Dr. Rapaport has authored 68 peer-reviewed papers on a wide range of dermatological topics, including psoriasis, silicone-related complications, patch testing, sunscreens, skin infections, and skin tumors. He has delivered 83 invited lectures at medical conferences and serves as a consultant to 41 law firms, offering expert testimony on complex dermatologic cases. His career spans more than five decades—bridging eras of medicine and generations of patients.

Despite curing countless patients by removing steroids entirely, and his stellar credentials and lengthy experience, his warnings have largely been ignored by the dermatology establishment. Imagine standing in a room full of experts, holding proof of a danger, only to be waved off as an outlier. That is Dr. Rapaport's reality.

When I asked Dr. Rapaport about being shunned, **he described a typical incident**. He told me about participating in a dermatology email group where colleagues traded advice on cases, billing, and policies. When he began responding to their many posts about red, rash-covered patients—classic TSA scenarios—by offering diagnosis, explanations, and treatment suggestions, the reaction was harsh. "They vilified me," he said, "and even tried to shut me down." Only when the group's director stepped in was he able to continue. **For him, it was a clear example of how many doctors respond with anger when their favorite drug is questioned. "Some of them were so proud to say that they give forty to sixty Kenalog (steroids) shots a week, and have done this for years."**

Dr. Rapaport is ridiculed, sidelined, and dismissed by peers who cannot fathom that their trusted go-to remedy might be the root of suffering. Still, he keeps going. Not for praise. Not for profit.

But because he knows he is right. And because patient after patient walks out of his office, finally healed.

And the truth? Dr. Rapaport doesn't have to do this. He could fade comfortably into retirement. He has already achieved professional success, having built a successful and reputable Beverly Hills dermatology practice.

But instead of coasting, he turns his attention to the people who are most ignored and misunderstood—those suffering in silence from steroid addiction.

His motivation isn't glory. It is duty and healing.

Dr. Rapaport often references the painful letters he receives from desperate patients—their skin oozing, their minds unraveling, their families in disbelief. He compares them to the letters received by "Miss Lonelyhearts," a fictional newspaper columnist from the 1930s. But these cries for help are all too real.

And he answers them. Thousands of times over decades. He says he still gets more than 500 emails a year.

For those most severely affected, Dr. Rapaport offers more than just validation. He provides hope, a plan, and often the only hand-holding support they will find. He tracks their recovery meticulously. He works with compassion and realism—never sugarcoating the path ahead, but always affirming there is light at the end of the tunnel.

He is maligned, misunderstood, and underestimated. Yet he never stops showing up—for his patients, for the truth, and for the future of medicine. He is still seeing patients, still taking new cases, and still urging the world to listen.

Dr. Rapaport is a rare kind of hero. Not flashy. Not self-serving. Just a brilliant mind with a compassionate heart who refuses to stay silent.

The loneliness of his path cannot be overstated. For decades, he has borne the weight of knowledge the world doesn't want. But for every patient he helps, for every life he saves from the grip of a false cure, he is more than a doctor. He is a light in the fog.

And for me, he was the first voice to say: *You are not crazy. You are not alone. You can heal. Now, let me show you how.*

He is not the first doctor to carry such a burden. History is filled with physicians who saw what others refused to see—and suffered for it because of medical dogma.

Medical Dogma Case Study #1: He Asked Doctors to Wash Their Hands

How a simple act of hygiene could have saved thousands—if only medicine had listened.

In the 1840s, Ignaz Semmelweis, a Hungarian physician, was haunted by the high maternal death rates in European hospitals. While doctors moved freely from autopsies to birthing rooms without washing their hands, women were dying from what was called "childbed fever"—a condition no one could explain.

Semmelweis saw what others refused to see. He hypothesized that invisible particles—what we now know as bacteria—were being transferred from corpses to living mothers. His solution was simple: doctors must wash their hands with chlorinated lime before delivering babies.

The result was revolutionary: maternal death rates plummeted. Yet the medical establishment responded not with gratitude, but with hostility. His peers were insulted by the suggestion that their hands were causing harm. The idea of "invisible contagion" was ridiculed as unscientific. Semmelweis was eventually ousted from his hospital position, labeled unstable, and confined to an asylum— where he died at 47, beaten by guards, and likely from sepsis, the very infection he had tried to prevent.

Fast forward 150 years, and the parallels to Dr. Marvin Rapaport are unmistakable. In a field saturated with blind trust in topical steroids, Rapaport sees something deeply troubling. Patients aren't just failing to improve—they are deteriorating. Their skin is thinning, their rashes are spreading, their suffering is deepening. And yet, the prescription pad keeps churning out more potent corticosteroids. Like Semmelweis, Rapaport connects the dots and sounds the alarm: the treatment itself is becoming the disease.

And just like Semmelweis, his warnings are met with dismissal and denial. The dermatology establishment, bound by convention, is unwilling to believe that their go-to treatment could be harming patients. His peer-reviewed research, his clinical success stories, even the visible recoveries of thousands of suffering patients aren't enough. He is brushed aside. Not with scientific refutation—but with silence.

Medical Dogma Case Study #2: The Doctor Who Drank Bacteria

When ridicule blocked the truth, he swallowed the proof—and changed medicine forever.

If Semmelweis showed how dogma crushed truth in the 1800s, Barry Marshall proved in the 1980s that even in the modern age, medicine still punishes those who see what others refuse to see.

Marshall, an Australian gastroenterologist, began to question one of medicine's most accepted truths: that stomach ulcers were caused by stress, acid, and lifestyle. For decades, patients were told to avoid spicy foods, take antacids, or even undergo stomach surgery. Ulcers were framed as a personality flaw—the disease of the anxious, the uptight, the Type A.

But Marshall and his colleague Robin Warren kept finding the same microscopic culprit in ulcer patients—a spiral-shaped **bacterium** later named *Helicobacter pylori*. Marshall proposed the unthinkable: ulcers were not a psychological condition or a stress reaction at all. They were an infection.

The response from the medical establishment was swift and scornful. Senior doctors dismissed him as naïve. Journals rejected his papers. One reviewer sneered that his theory was "the medical equivalent of saying the Earth is flat." The idea that a simple bacterium could upend a billion-dollar ulcer industry built on antacids and surgeries was too threatening to entertain.

Frustrated, Marshall decided to prove his theory in the most dramatic way possible: he drank a glass of *H. pylori* himself. Within days he developed violent gastritis. His stomach lining inflamed, his breath reeked of sulfur, and his biopsies showed bacterial overgrowth. He had deliberately given himself the disease. Then, with a simple course of antibiotics, he cured it.

Acceptance was slow. For years, he was mocked, ignored, and shut out. But the evidence mounted, replication followed, and eventually, the medical world could no longer deny it. In 2005, Barry Marshall and Robin Warren were awarded the Nobel Prize in Medicine for proving that bacteria—not stress—caused ulcers.

These case studies reveal a timeless pattern in medicine: when truth collides with dogma, dogma fights back.

Like Rapaport, Marshall and Semmelweis weren't seeking fame; they simply followed the evidence and refused to look away. Marshall lived to see vindication. Semmelweis did not.

Like Semmelweis and Marshall, Dr. Rapaport never stops speaking up. These men weren't trying to be rebels. They were scientists with eyes wide open—and hearts rooted in duty. They saw what others missed. They noticed the patterns, listened to the patients, and followed the truth even when it cost them professionally. Semmelweis told doctors to wash their hands. Marshall said ulcers were caused by a bacterium. Rapaport tells them to put down the steroid cream.

And like Semmelweis and Marshall, Rapaport pays a price. His message is slow to gain traction. **His warnings remain inconve-**

nient for a system built on symptom suppression rather than root-cause resolution. But history has a way of circling back. Today, handwashing is a cornerstone of medical hygiene. Antibiotics are the standard cure for ulcers. And one day soon, the link between long-term steroid use and systemic harm will no longer be ignored.

History may not remember the accolades Dr. Rapaport doesn't receive—but it will remember the lives he saves.

Just as Semmelweis is now hailed as a pioneer of antiseptic medicine, and Marshall a Nobel Prize winner, Rapaport will one day be recognized as the doctor who exposed the false cure of topical steroids—before the world was ready to believe it. With the speed of information today, history seems to be catching up—and when it does, may Dr. Rapaport finally receive the recognition he has long deserved.

Dr. Marvin Rapaport stands as the elder statesman of this movement and the father of TSW. His groundbreaking research not only gave patients language for their suffering but also inspired physicians around the world to confront the harm caused by long-term steroid use and pursue their own clinical investigations. Just as the practice of law requires precedent to move forward, medicine requires precedent too. Without Dr. Rapaport's work, later physicians would have had little foundation on which to build—or to establish the proof the world needs about TSA.

We had awakened—not just me, but a pattern too big to ignore. The next step was clear: to prove it. To show that what we were living was not rare, not anecdotal, but epidemic.

It started with an itch. It became an awakening. Now it demands proof.

Publications by Marvin J. Rapaport on Red Skin Syndrome, Topical Steroid Addiction and Withdrawal

For further findings on these topics, see Appendix 2.

1. Rapaport MJ, Rapaport V. *Eyelid dermatitis to red face syndrome to cure: clinical experience in 100 cases.* J Am Acad Dermatol. 1999;41(3 Pt 1):435–442. doi:10.1016/S0190-9622(99)70118-0.

2. Rapaport MJ, Rapaport V. *Prolonged erythema after facial laser resurfacing or phenol peel secondary to corticosteroid addiction.* Dermatol Surg. 1999;25(10):781–784; discussion 785. doi:10.1046/j.1524-4725.1999.99097.x.

3. Rapaport MJ, Lebwohl M. *Corticosteroid addiction and withdrawal in the atopic: the red burning skin syndrome.* Clin Dermatol. 2003;21(3):201–214. doi:10.1016/S0738-081X(02)00365-6.

4. Rapaport MJ, Rapaport VH. *Serum nitric oxide levels in "red" patients: separating corticosteroid-addicted patients from those with chronic eczema.* Arch Dermatol. 2004;140(8):1013–1014. doi:10.1001/arFchderm.140.8.1013.

5. Rapaport MJ, Rapaport V. *The red skin syndromes: corticosteroid addiction and withdrawal.* Expert Rev Dermatol. 2006;1(4):547–561. doi:10.1586/17469872.1.4.547.

6. Rapaport MJ. *Rebound vasodilation from long-term topical corticosteroid use.* Arch Dermatol. 2007;143(2):268–269. doi:10.1001/archderm.143.2.268-b.

PART II

THE PROOF

CHAPTER FOUR

THE POSIT: PROVING THE CASE

CONSIDER THIS THE OPENING ARGUMENT: three chapters that lay out the proof no institution can ignore. The next three chapters in this section of the book are called Proof. Here we lay out the case. First, the central posits—the five claims this book intends to prove. Then, the global prevalence and evidence: numbers, symptoms, and stories that repeat with uncanny precision across continents. And finally, the trail of the creams themselves: how a drug born in promise as a miracle became a product pushed without caution, its risks hidden in plain sight.

Dr. Rapaport's story shows what one set of eyes, fully open, can see when everyone else looks away. But one doctor's courage—no matter how extraordinary—isn't enough to change a system. If this fight is going to be won, we have to prove the case so clearly that denial is no longer an option.

Now it is not just my story, not just Rachel's, not just Dr. Rapaport's patients. **It is our global story—backed by data, worldwide voices, and decades of evidence.** Before we go any further, I want you to know exactly what I intend to prove.

Posit #1 — TSW is real.

Topical Steroid Addiction and Withdrawal are real, documented conditions and have been for decades—recognized in medical literature, described by physicians across multiple countries, and visible in patient recoveries.

Posit #2 — Prevalence is far higher than admitted.

TSW potentially affects millions, including children, yet remains hidden by the absence of a diagnostic code, registry, or tracking system.

Posit #3 — The harm is real and preventable.

With better prescribing practices, informed consent, safer alternatives, and honest warnings, countless cases of TSW and its damaging effects could be avoided.

Posit #4 — Patterns match globally.

From Tokyo to Kolkata, Sydney to Los Angeles, the stories and symptoms match too closely to dismiss and they are different from the patterns of worsening eczema.

Posit #5 — The medical establishment has ignored warning signs for decades.

Despite published studies, photographic evidence, and patient testimonies that span generations, institutions have chosen silence, denial, and reputational protection over truth.

But these five points are only part of the story.

The most glaring—and almost irrefutable—truth is this: Topical Steroid Withdrawal isn't rare, accidental, or mysterious. It's the predictable, pharmacologic consequence of how these drugs are prescribed, labeled, and sold.

Topical Steroid Withdrawal isn't rare, accidental, or mysterious. It is the predict-able result of how these drugs alter skin physiology, blood vessels, and immune function. When they are used repeatedly, over time, the body adapts—just as it does with any dependency-forming drug. Addiction and withdrawal isn't a rare complication; it is the expected outcome of the very treatment guidelines patients are told to follow. The suffering that follows is not simply a flare of eczema, but a preventable iatrogenic syndrome with clear and unmistakable hallmarks that set it apart from eczema itself.

—Dr. Marvin J. Rapaport, Clinical Professor of Dermatology and Medicine, UCLA

Not everyone who uses topical steroids will develop full-blown TSW—just as not every smoker develops lung cancer.

But the risk is baked into the product, and the harm is multiplied by the way it's used. The medical establishment knows how dependence works. They have decades of pharmacologic evidence. Which means this isn't a mystery illness, or even an accident.

It is the natural, foreseeable consequence of a system that tells patients these drugs are safe for routine use, offers no long-term safety monitoring, and hides the withdrawal risk in plain sight.

Tobacco Twin

If this sounds extreme, remember: the tobacco industry used the exact same playbook.

For decades, cigarette makers had internal research showing nicotine was addictive, that smoking caused cancer, and that their product could kill. They didn't just ignore the evidence—they buried it, discredited the scientists, and paid for their own "research" to sow doubt. They rolled out marketing campaigns with slogans like "More doctors smoke Camels" and placed smiling physicians in ads to assure the public there was nothing to fear.

When the lawsuits came, they hid behind a familiar line: "Not everyone who smokes gets sick."

Technically true—and completely misleading. Not everyone who smokes gets cancer, but everyone who smokes becomes addicted. And every cigarette damages the body, whether it ends in a tumor or not.

Tobacco and TSW Parallels

Not everyone will develop the most extreme form of withdrawal—but every patient who uses them long-term is at risk of dependency. Every application alters skin function. Every prolonged course raises the odds that stopping will unleash symptoms the system has no plan to manage.

And just as tobacco companies fought for decades to keep the public in the dark, the dermatology establishment and pharmaceutical industry now cling to the same talking points:

- "It's rare."
- "It's not proven."
- "The benefits outweigh the risks."

Skeptics often tell us the same thing: "You don't have the science." That's why this section exists. These posits are the science all in one place—documented patterns, global prevalence, pharmacology, clinical papers and decades of overlooked evidence.

But here's the truth: dermatology doesn't have the science to deny it either.

> *The most baffling part is how definitive experts sound against TSW despite their complete lack of research.*
>
> —Dr. Ian Myles, Principal Investigator of the Epithelial Therapeutics Unit at National Institutes of Health, National Institutes of Allergy and Infectious Diseases

That is the vacuum this part of the book begins to fill. TSW doctors and researchers have been at work for decades. Dermatology "experts" are going off studies published over 70 years ago done on less potent applications in insufficient test populations. The TSW evidence is here, the patterns are global, and denial can no longer hide behind the claim of "no science."

CHAPTER FIVE

GLOBAL PRESENCE AND PREVALENCE

‖‖

It's Only Rare If You Refuse to Measure It.

BEFORE WE TALK ABOUT THE STAGGERING global numbers—let's talk about Flint, Michigan. In 2014, officials in Flint changed the city's water supply to cut costs. Almost immediately, residents complained of rashes, strange smells, and brown tap water. Children began showing signs of lead poisoning. But when parents raised concerns, they were told not to worry. That the water was safe. That lead poisoning was rare.

Except it wasn't.

The truth was far worse. Flint's pipes were corroding. Lead levels were spiking. But there was no formal surveillance system. No lead screening protocol. No mechanism for recognizing or reporting what was happening. And so, for months—what was actually a public health emergency was labeled "rare."[1]

Because no one was looking.

You cannot call something rare if you've never measured it.

You cannot measure what you've never named.

And you cannot name what your system refuses to see.

This is exactly what's happening with Topical Steroid Withdrawal (TSW).[2]

There's no diagnostic code. No registry. No long-term safety data. No tracking system. TSW is not formally recognized in most medical training, not reimbursed by insurers, and not routinely recorded in dermatology databases.[3]

So when patients burn, flake, ooze, or see their health unravel after continually using, or stopping steroid creams, the system shrugs: must be a flare of eczema, or—if they are feeling generous—a rare reaction to the drug.[2]

But how do you measure withdrawal from a drug the system swears isn't addictive? Until we track it—honestly, transparently, and globally—calling TSW rare is not medicine. It's manufactured ignorance.[4]

Now, if Jane Austen were alive today and writing about dermatology instead of the English gentry, she might have called this chapter *Pride and Prejudice* (instead of presence and prevalence). Pride—because too many doctors have let ego eclipse evidence, brushing off the mounting voices of suffering patients as exaggeration or internet hysteria. And prejudice—because the dogma runs deep. If it's not in their textbook or backed by their society's stamp of approval, it must not exist.

But we're not here to rehash 19th-century literature—we're here to prove what we laid out in Chapter 4:

- TSW is real.
- Its prevalence is far higher than admitted.
- The harm is preventable.
- The patterns repeat across continents.
- And the medical establishment has ignored the warning signs for decades.

One diligent dermatologist in Japan set out to give us the data that could no longer be denied.

Japan: Dr. Fukaya's Data-Driven Warning

While most of the world's dermatology establishments were side-stepping the issue of TSW—or worse, denying it outright—one man decided to do what no one else had dared: try to officially measure it.[2]

Enter Dr. Mototsugu Fukaya, a Japanese dermatologist who didn't only believe the patients—he studied them, like Dr. Rapaport had, albeit decades later. While the National Eczema Association (NEA) tiptoed around the subject with vague references to anecdotal reports, Dr. Fukaya rolled up his sleeves, dug into clinical patterns, and published a paper that delivered exactly what the world needed: prevalence data.

In his 2014 article, *Topical Steroid Addiction in Atopic Dermatitis,* **published in** *Drug, Healthcare and Patient Safety,* **Dr. Fukaya estimated that approximately 12% of adult patients diagnosed with atopic dermatitis in Japan were actually suffering from Topical Steroid Addiction.**[5] Twelve percent. That's more than one in ten. And yet, at the time of publication—and even today in many circles—TSA was still being treated as a fringe theory or an internet myth.

Dr. Fukaya didn't pull this number from thin air. His estimate was rooted in years of clinical observation, case reviews, and an honest willingness to confront what was happening every day in his presence. He described patients whose conditions worsened not in spite of their prescribed treatment, but because of it.[2]

Individuals who applied steroid creams religiously, only to find that their rashes spread, their skin became hypersensitive, and—most tellingly—they developed a burning sensation that classic eczema could not explain.[2]

He laid out the key clinical distinction, the same as Dr. Rapaport had earlier, another diagnostic north star for doctors who dared to see the difference: eczema itches; steroid addiction burns when patients are becoming addicted and then itches more deeply than eczema when they stop using the medications.

And it wasn't just a semantic difference. Fukaya's patients experienced widespread rebound erythema (redness, or darkening in pigmented skin), hypersensitivity to touch and temperature, and inflammation that radiated far beyond the original treatment areas. These symptoms occurred only after stopping the steroids—a classic withdrawal pattern, not a flare-up.

This condition had been given a name. It had been given a description. But most importantly, now, he gave it a number.[2]

That Number Came at a Cost

We've talked about the pain of patients. We've talked about the emotional burden of caregivers and the strain on spouses. But what we haven't talked about yet is the pain carried by doctors like Dr. Fukaya—those who dare to speak against their profession's dogma and pay the price for it.[4]

Working within Japan's National Hospital System, where topical steroids were freely and widely dispensed under universal healthcare, Dr. Fukaya had a unique perspective and saw firsthand how widespread addiction had become. He spent more than a decade documenting and photographing patient cases, ultimately writing a 35-chapter monograph on TSA, with multiple time-lapsed photos, that captured the stark realities of this condition. And yet, despite the depth of his research, he found himself ignored—or worse, dismissed—by many of his own colleagues.

The weight of being unheard took a toll. Dr. Fukaya has shared this with me in an email, and again openly in his public blog, how this professional isolation led to deep frustration, burnout, and depression. But he found temporary support by meeting someone who had been a great inspiration to him: Dr. Marvin Rapaport. In

2010, Dr. Fukaya visited Rapaport in his Beverly Hills office, where they spoke for an hour and Fukaya presented his printed book filled with the photos and histories of TSA patients he had treated. It was a meaningful meeting of two physicians who would go on to shape the global understanding of TSA. Dr. Fukaya's work remains one of the most critical scientific contributions in the field of TSW, serving as both a warning and a roadmap for those willing to look past the myths.

Let's talk numbers. Because while the medical establishment may wave away stories as "anecdotal," it becomes a lot harder to dismiss the math.

Apply Dr. Fukaya's 12% TSA prevalence estimate to the adult global eczema population, which can be conservatively estimated at 2.5 percent of 6 billion adults in the world, giving eczema patients a number of 150 million. So if 150 million adults have eczema, then 12% of that is 18 million adults at risk for TSW. That math becomes chilling.

That's over 18 million adults worldwide who may be unknowingly experiencing drug-induced damage to their skin and health while continuing to follow doctor's orders.[2] This number does not include children who have a much higher rate of eczema.

And for those who might argue that Japan's healthcare model makes the data irrelevant elsewhere, it's worth pointing out: topical corticosteroids are just as ubiquitous—if not more so—in Western countries. In the United States alone, 31.6 million people have some form of eczema, and 16.5 million adults are diagnosed with atopic dermatitis.[9] These individuals almost universally receive topical steroids as part of their treatment plan.[10]

Moreover, usage patterns show long-term exposure is the norm, not the exception. In one recent cohort, the average duration of steroid use was found to be 15.3 years in adults and 3.6 years in children.[11]

Tens of Millions of Children at Risk

Children make up one of the largest—and most vulnerable—populations affected by topical steroid use. Globally, 20-25% of children suffer from atopic dermatitis, compared to roughly 2.5% of adults. With a 12 percent prevalence rate, that is 48-60 million children at risk for TSW.[39, 40]

That means more than a billion people worldwide are living with eczema at any given time. And when you apply Dr. Mototsugu Fukaya's cautious but credible estimate—that 12% of patients with atopic dermatitis are actually experiencing topical steroid addiction (TSA)—the numbers become staggering.[31]

By the total math:

- Global population (2025): ~8 billion.[41]
- Children (~25%): ~2 billion
- AD prevalence 20–25% → 400–500 million children with AD[39]
- 12% with TSA → ~48–60 million children[31]
- Adults (~75%): ~6 billion
- AD prevalence: ~2.5% → ~150 million adults with AD[40]
- 12% with TSA → ~18 million adults[31]

Total estimate:
As many as 66–78 million people worldwide—adults and children combined—may be living with topical steroid addiction or withdrawal.

Yet here's the uncomfortable truth: there have been no formal clinical studies on TSA or TSW in children. This means millions of children are using a potent, hormone-altering drug on a developing body—sometimes for years—without the benefit of long-term safety data or diagnostic protocols for withdrawal syndromes.[4]

Their suffering is invisible not because it doesn't exist, but because it has never been formally studied.

Patients are starting to speak up. In a 2024 survey published in *JAAD*, 71.8% of topical steroid users said they believed steroids had damaged their skin, with many reporting symptoms consistent with withdrawal, including burning, spreading redness, and dependency-like patterns of use.[12]

These numbers demand attention. Not denial. Not deflection.

If TSA were rare, the math wouldn't check out. But it does. If TSA weren't real, we wouldn't see the same burning, spreading, treatment-resistant patterns documented across multiple continents, thousands of patient testimonies, and decades of case reports.[2]

And if TSA weren't being actively ignored by the medical establishment, doctors like Dr. Fukaya and Dr. Rapaport wouldn't have suffered professional isolation and silence for trying to expose it.[4]

Pen Pals

Anecdotally, I should add something personal here. Over the years, Dr. Fukaya and I became pen pals, exchanging emails as I tried to make sense of the TSA landscape. In one of those messages, **he confided to me that he actually believed the prevalence of topical steroid addiction was much higher than 12%**. But, as he explained, after being berated and dismissed by his peers in Japan, he felt he needed to start with a conservative number—one that could be easily shown and would not ignite another storm of ridicule. As we've seen in this chapter, he had already taken more than his share of arrows for daring to name and number what others refused to see.

Even Dr. Fukaya's conservative research numbers sent a shockwave through the dermatological world. In Japan, the warning signs weren't just theoretical—they were visible, measurable, and growing. And if the patterns he documented seemed familiar to patients in the West, they were already being lived, daily, in other corners of the world.

Now, we turn to the most populated country on Earth—India— where the collision of pharmaceutical access, cultural beauty ideals, and regulatory delay has created one of the most widespread and dangerous hotbeds of topical steroid misuse in the world.

India: Where Commerce Meets Culture

But first, meet Meera.

She didn't think she was ugly. She just thought she was... too dark.

In her twenties, Meera* (name changed for privacy) was bright, ambitious, and newly graduated with a degree in psychology. She dreamed of modeling one day—maybe even appearing on television. But every time she looked in the mirror, one thought whispered louder than the rest: her skin tone was holding her back.

It wasn't shame exactly. It was something more insidious. A belief, passed down subtly through generations, media, and offhand comments. That lighter skin meant a better chance. That fair was beautiful. That dark was not.

So Meera began using a fairness cream. She applied it before bed, after waking up, between errands, and again at night.

"It's like a drug," she once said. "If I don't put it on, I feel like I'll go darker."

No one warned her that the cream—sold innocently over the counter and marketed with pastel labels and smiling models—might contain a potent corticosteroid. No one told her she might become dependent. That her skin might thin, burn, or erupt. That this wasn't just cosmetic.

"Asian people don't think a dark-skinned girl can be beautiful," she said. "I think that started when England colonized India."

Her words echoed far beyond her own experience. They reflect a deeper truth across modern India—a truth that has turned cultural insecurity into a pharmaceutical cash cow, and skincare into steroid exposure.

Why TSA Is So Prevalent in India

India's topical steroid crisis didn't arrive overnight. It built up, quietly, over decades—driven by underregulated pharmacies, powerful marketing, and a deeply entrenched preference for lighter skin.[2]

Over-the-Counter Access

Until just a few years ago, high-potency topical corticosteroids—like clobetasol, mometasone, and betamethasone—were widely available without a prescription.[13] Often disguised as anti-itch or whitening creams, they were sold under charming names and misleading labels. A 2021 IADVL report documented over 100 irrational fixed-dose steroid combinations in Indian pharmacies, many blending steroids with antifungals or antibiotics—creating products both harmful and medically nonsensical.[2]

Fairness Culture and Cosmetic Cover-Up

In a society where lighter skin still opens doors—socially, professionally, and matrimonially—"fairness creams" are a billion-dollar industry. Many users apply them daily, unaware they're using a hormone-altering medication. One study found that over 70% of users didn't know their fairness cream contained a steroid.[14] They thought they were moisturizing. Instead, they were medicating.

Misinformation and Self-Medication

In much of India, topical steroids are recommended not by doctors, but by friends, relatives, or local shopkeepers. And when withdrawal symptoms appear—burning, redness, flares—users assume it's their skin, not the drug. So they reapply. Again and again.[4]

Regulatory Delays

Although the Indian government banned 328 irrational fixed-dose combinations in 2018, enforcement has been inconsistent. Many of the creams are still sold under the counter, online, or under different names. For every product pulled, another takes its place.

India's Medical Truth-Tellers

Dr. Koushik Lahiri – The Terminologist

A respected Kolkata-based dermatologist, Dr. Lahiri was among the first to give the condition a name: *Topical Steroid Damaged/ Dependent Face (TSDF).*[15] Once he named it, he couldn't unsee it. Patient after patient walked into his clinic—young women with thinning skin, depigmentation, scarring—and all with the same silent addiction to fairness creams.

In 2007, he co-authored a proposal to IADVL that became the foundation for India's steroid ban a decade later.[16] His work earned him the *Members Making a Difference Award* from the American Academy of Dermatology—a rare honor for an Indian physician.

Dr. Rajetha Damisetty – The Enforcer

As Chair of IADVL's Task Force Against Topical Steroid Abuse, Dr. Damisetty has pushed for clinical consistency and public educa-tion. She's led the development of treatment protocols, awareness initiatives, and position papers that challenge both corporate irresponsibility and clinical complacency.[17] She has warned that once the skin is dependent, it's already late in the game—what matters most is preventing that first unnecessary prescription or application.[2]

Dr. Arijit Coondoo – The Strategist

Behind much of India's early momentum was Dr. Coondoo, who co-authored the 2007 proposal with Lahiri.[16] His academic rigor and policy advocacy helped validate what many doctors saw anecdotally but hadn't yet defined. He framed the crisis in language that could reach regulators and institutional bodies—an essential step in forcing national acknowledgment.

Dr. Sandipan Dhar – The Child Defender

No one has done more to protect India's children from the harm of steroids than Dr. Dhar. As the country's foremost pediatric dermatologist and President of the Indian Society for Pediatric Dermatology, and Founding President of the Society of Eczema Studies, he has published more than 200 papers, authored the *Colour Atlas and Synopsis of Paediatric Dermatology*,[18] and contributed to global eczema research through his role on the International Eczema Council.

But it's his warnings about early exposure that carry the most urgency. He has spoken of children so sensitized from prolonged steroid use that they flinch when touched—of young patients whose confidence is shattered not by eczema, but by the after-effects of the drugs meant to help them.[2]

These doctors don't carry protest signs or sue corporations. They publish. They warn. They teach. They refuse to stay silent. In India—a country navigating one of the largest unregulated steroid crises with the world's largest population—they are the line between misinformation and reform. If the nation is to climb out of this pharmaceutical quicksand, it will be because of voices like theirs.[4]

These doctors may never appear on a global stage. Their names won't trend on social media. But inside clinics and conference rooms, they've ignited a shift in how India understands skin—and the drugs meant to treat it. And India isn't alone. From Tokyo to

Kolkata, the evidence is mounting. The stories are multiplying. And if there's one thing that unites them, it's this: the damage doesn't stop at borders.[2]

Which brings us to another continent entirely.

Australia: Stuck in Neutral

Australia is a land known for sun, surf, and skin-consciousness. But even here—in a country with high dermatological literacy and a regulated healthcare system—the truth about topical steroids has been harder to swallow than expected.[2]

In June 2024, *Dermatology Republic* ran an article that neatly illustrated the problem with calling something "extremely rare" when there's no agreed-upon name, no tracking, and no diagnostic code. In it, Australian dermatology leaders acknowledged that topical steroid withdrawal (TSW) exists—but insisted it was "very rare" and urged patients not to stop treatment without medical supervision. The piece framed TSW as a possible complication of "overuse" rather than the result of standard, guideline-based prescribing. Post-steroid symptoms were often recast as "rebound eczema," and the need for further research was buried under warnings against deviating from conventional treatment.[19]

It's the same logic problem we saw at the start of this chapter: calling something rare when you've made it almost impossible to measure.[2] And yet, "extremely rare" starts to look like willful blindness when you stack it against the global publications and in-country work of just one Australian GP who has spent more than a decade publishing almost a dozen studies on TSW—research from her own clinic.

That doctor is Dr. Belinda Sheary, a general practitioner. While most of Australia's medical establishment has kept its head down, Sheary has quietly been documenting the truth for years. Her 2016 primer for general practitioners laid out the syndrome's hallmark signs—burning pain, widespread redness, hypersensitivity—and warned that it could arise from guideline-based prescribing, not just obvious overuse.[20]

Sheary went further. In 2018, she published a 55-patient adult cohort, proposing diagnostic features like the "red sleeve" and "elephant wrinkles" that have since become touchstones for patient and clinician recognition.[21] Her 2019 case series of ten children tracked recovery over months to years, showing that many improved once the drugs were stopped.[22] And in 2021, she followed 24 adults for two years post-cessation, finding that while withdrawal was initially devastating, most saw significant quality-of-life gains over time.[23]

Taken together, her work dismantles the "extremely rare" narrative by showing consistent patterns across age groups, settings, and continents. Yet despite this contribution, Sheary's findings have not broken through to the broader Australian dermatology conversation. They remain tucked into academic journals while the public narrative continues to frame TSW as an anomaly—proof that even when the evidence exists, it takes more than data to move a medical culture entrenched in denial.

The only identifiable source attempting to address TSW is Eczema Support Australia, which has partnered with a few supportive healthcare professionals to develop educational resources for people impacted by eczema and TSW.[24] However, like you'll learn in a future chapter, patient advocacy organizations are often steered by medical advisors' agendas and pharma dollars.[2]

On the mainstream media front, the silence was broken—at least briefly—when Jordan Hendey, a young man from Western Australia, went public with his story. Prescribed topical steroids from the age of two, Jordan's skin gradually thinned over the years until stopping them triggered a cascade of agonizing symptoms. He described the pain as "like thousands of papercuts all over your body" and the flaking so severe that his clothes and sheets looked dusted with snow. Doctors told him it was "just a flare." Desperate, he traveled to Bangkok for treatment—because no one in Australia seemed willing to guide him through withdrawal.[25]

Jordan's courage and persistence forced attention on the issue. In the wake of media coverage, the Australasian College of Dermatologists (ACD), the Royal Australian College of General Practitioners (RACGP), and Eczema Support Australia issued formal acknowledgment of TSW as a rare but real reaction. Still, his case remains one of the only widely reported examples in the country—a lone voice in a medical landscape that continues to treat the syndrome as an outlier.[2]

While some Australian research has examined the outcomes of patients stopping long-term steroid use—finding widely varied recovery times—these studies have not yet sparked the kind of systemic awareness or advocacy seen elsewhere. Without strong public voices, Australia's patients are left to navigate withdrawal largely in the shadows, told their suffering is "extremely rare" while their bodies tell a different story.

The United Kingdom: Rising Authority, Dr. George Moncrieff

And while this chapter has focused mainly on Japan, India, and Australia, in the United Kingdom—a country we have yet to fully explore—a crucial voice has quietly emerged.

Dr. George Moncrieff, a retired GP and former chair of the Dermatology Council for England, has suggested that as many as one in ten patients with persistent or severe eczema could actually be experiencing topical steroid withdrawal—not just a flare or rebound.[26] His 10 percent estimate offers one important indicator of the scale of the problem in the UK, and signals a growing willingness to name what has been dismissed for too long.[4]

Dr. Moncrieff is also a member of the ITSAN Advisory Council and Medical Advisory Board, lending his clinical credibility to the global effort to recognize and address TSW.[2]

The UK section will be brief here, because later we'll explore in depth how Britain has become a world leader in TSW advocacy and activism. Unlike other countries—where TSW is dismissed, denied, or spoken of in whispers—the UK is the only place where patients are mobilizing as true activists. They are not just talking about TSW; they are protesting in the streets, pushing media coverage, demanding recognition, and winning label changes. Where Japan measured, India warned, and Australia hesitated, the UK is mobilizing.

From the UK to across the pond in the United States where we met the original doctor who saw *the presence, the prevalence, the patterns* and spoke up, but he was alone, until recently. It took decades before someone joined Dr. Rapaport's voice. That someone is Dr. Peter Lio.

The USA: A New Voice, Dr. Peter Lio

TSW is starting to go mainstream. At the Revolutionizing Atopic Dermatitis (RAD) Conference in 2025, Dr. Peter Lio, Clinical Assistant Professor of Dermatology and Pediatrics at Northwestern University's Feinberg School of Medicine, took the stage alongside two colleagues to address TSW head-on. Unlike many in his field, he acknowledged it openly, described its distinct clinical features, and—most importantly—called on his peers to listen to patients.[27] The following section is paraphrased from his presentation, which can be found in full at HCPLive.

Dr. Lio explained. "I meet clinicians who say, 'I don't think it's a real entity' or 'I think it's no different than atopic dermatitis,' but I try to convey some of the symptoms that are different and, most importantly, even if you don't acknowledge it or accept it, I think we should still hear our patients out."[27]

This alone marked a major shift. For decades, patients reporting withdrawal were dismissed. But here was a dermatologist, on stage, not only validating their voices but showing his colleagues that humility is strength, not weakness.

Dr. Lio also explained why so many physicians push back—and why patient testimony feels threatening:

"Patients often come in telling us that they have this, and that is a big reversal for dermatology. The patient says, 'I think I have TSW,' and we're not built for that. We know a lot more than the patients do, so I feel like it's a weird reaction to be threatened, but I get it. It feels threatening, like they're kind of trying to usurp you."[27]

Here, Lio named what so many patients have felt but couldn't articulate: that our voices disrupt the traditional hierarchy of medicine. For some doctors, this feels like a threat to their expertise. But as Lio reminds us, it shouldn't.

He has even reassured his own patients directly:

"I can reassure them, 'You may not know this, but I'm a TSW person and I've written about it.... Usually when I say that, their shoulders drop, they relax, and they smile."[27]

For patients, after years of being told "this condition does not exist," those words are a breath of oxygen. Dr. Lio gave not only recognition, but also an explanation for the wall we so often hit in exam rooms. He showed his peers that listening to patients is not capitulation—it is clinical evidence in action.

Posits Reinforced by Dr. Lio's Testimony:

- TSW is real.
- TSW presents a different clinical pattern from eczema.
- TSW is prevalent enough that patients are now bringing the diagnosis to their doctors.
- Patient testimony is evidence that deserves respect, not dismissal.
- Doctors can change their minds—and when they do, patients feel seen.

We've now seen that the numbers, the symptoms, and the stories are consistent across continents.[2] This is not a local quirk, a rare reaction, or an online echo chamber—it is a predictable outcome of a treatment that has been marketed, prescribed, and sold the same way for generations.

The Science Speaks

This is where the proof and prevalence become undeniable—the science speaks.

- 34 studies documenting cases of TSW across the medical literature, pulled together in systematic reviews.[28]
- 320+ pediatric cases of steroid-related dermatitis consistent with withdrawal reported in clinical reviews.[29]
- 1,479 documented cases of TSW described across two systematic reviews, consolidating global case reports.[28]
- 1,200+ additional cases reported in published case series and reports.[30]
- 12% prevalence among adults with atopic dermatitis in Japan—translating to tens of millions affected worldwide.[31]
- A multinational survey found 79% of adults and 43% of caregivers reported TSW-like symptoms.[32]
- An Australian clinic cohort tracked dozens of adult patients with confirmed TSW over years of follow-up.[33]
- The UK's regulator, MHRA, has formally acknowledged TSW via Yellow Card reporting, logging dozens of "probable" and "possible" cases and issuing public guidance.[34]
- TSW has been documented on six continents—a true global epidemic.

The Global Proof

TSW is not rare. It is global—documented on every continent but Antarctica. In Asia, prevalence data from Japan and widespread misuse in India confirm the scale of the crisis.[31] In Europe, the UK has become a proving ground, with estimates from clinicians and acknowledgement by regulators.[26] Across North America, decades of peer-reviewed papers, survey data, and patient testimonies have pointed to the same patterns.[36] In Australia, Dr. Belinda Sheary's clinical studies, along with media reports, have forced the issue into public view.[20] In South America, cases from Brazil and Argentina have been captured in systematic reviews.[28] And in Africa, reports from Nigeria, South Africa, and beyond reveal the damage of steroid-laced skin-lightening creams.[38] Together, the evidence is irrefutable: TSW is not a rare complication but a global epidemic.

How did a class of drugs with clear addictive potential and devastating withdrawal effects become the first-line treatment for one of the most common skin conditions on Earth?

How did we reach a point where doctors can see the evidence in front of them yet still reach for the prescription pad without a warning?

And how did doctors come to believe that these creams were harmless—safe enough for infants, over-the-counter use, and years of daily application?

To answer that, we need to rewind the tape. We need to follow the path from discovery to distribution to dependence—the "miracle cream" story the pharmaceutical industry still wants you to believe.

Because until we understand the history, we cannot change the future.

IIIIIIIIIIIIIIIIIIIIIIIIIIIIIIIIIIIIIIIIIIIIIIIIIIIIIIIIIIIIIIIIIIIIIIIIIIIIIIIIIIIIIIIIIIIIIIIIIIIIIIIIIIIIIIIIIIIIIIIIIII

References

1. Hanna-Attisha M, LaChance J, Sadler RC, Schnepp AC. (2016). Elevated blood lead levels in children associated with the Flint drinking water crisis: A spatial analysis of risk and public health response. *American Journal of Public Health*, 106(2):283–290. [PubMed 26691115]

2. Posits referenced throughout this chapter (Posit #1 – TSW is real; Posit #2 – Prevalence is far higher than admitted).

3. Lindberg I, et al. (2021). Topical steroid withdrawal: A survey of international patients. *Dermatitis*, 32(5):301–309.

4. Posit #5 – The medical establishment has ignored warning signs for decades.

5. Fukaya M. (2014). Topical steroid addiction in atopic dermatitis. *Drug, Healthcare and Patient Safety*, 6:131–138. [PMC4171913]

6. Thyssen JP, et al. (2019). Atopic dermatitis: Global prevalence and risk factors. *British Journal of Dermatology*, 181(5):954–960.

7. NIH Clinical Guidelines. (2015). Atopic dermatitis: Treatment guidelines. *NCBI Bookshelf*.

8. Smith SD, et al. (2018). Patterns of topical corticosteroid use and factors associated with prolonged therapy in adults with atopic dermatitis. *Journal of the American Academy of Dermatology (JAAD)*, 79(2):294–301.

9. National Eczema Association. (2021). *Eczema Statistics*.

10. JAMA Dermatology. (2021). Prevalence and treatment patterns in atopic dermatitis: A U.S. survey analysis.

11. Smith SD, et al. (2022). Long-term use of topical corticosteroids in adults and children with atopic dermatitis: A cohort study. *JAAD*, 86(6):1232–1240.

12. Silverberg JI, et al. (2024). Patient-reported harm from topical steroids: A multinational survey. *JAAD*. [PMID: 39220458]

13. Indian Association of Dermatologists, Venereologists and Leprologists (IADVL). (2021). Task Force Against Topical Steroid Abuse: Report on irrational steroid combinations.

14. Pollock BH, Thomas KS, et al. (2021). Harmful skin-lightening products containing corticosteroids: A global public health issue. *British Journal of Dermatology*, 185(6):1087–1095.

15. Lahiri K. (2016). Topical steroid damaged/dependent face (TSDF): An entity of cutaneous pharmacodependence. *Indian Journal of Dermatology*, 61(3):265–272.

16. Lahiri K, Coondoo A. (2007). Proposal to IADVL for awareness on steroid misuse. *Indian Journal of Dermatology, Venereology and Leprology*.

17. Damisetty R, et al. (2021). IADVL Task Force Against Topical Steroid Abuse: Position paper. *Indian Dermatology Online Journal*.

18. Dhar S. (2019). *Colour Atlas and Synopsis of Pediatric Dermatology*, 2nd ed. Jaypee Brothers Medical Publishers.

19. *Dermatology Republic.* (2024, June 12). Call for calm over topical steroid withdrawal reports.

20. Sheary B, et al. (2016). Topical steroid withdrawal: A primer for general practitioners. *Australian Family Physician*, 45(8):584–587.

21. Sheary B, et al. (2018). Topical steroid withdrawal: Adult cohort study of 55 patients. *Australasian Journal of Dermatology*, 59(2):91–97.

22. Sheary B, et al. (2019). Topical steroid withdrawal in children: A case series of 10 patients. *Clinical and Experimental Dermatology*, 44(7):787–793.

23. Sheary B, et al. (2021). Topical steroid withdrawal: A two-year prospective study of quality of life in adults ceasing long-term use. *Dermatitis*, 32(6):406–414.

24. Eczema Support Australia. (2023). *Educational resources on eczema and TSW*. [Organization website].

25. ABC News Australia. (2024, June 12). Jordan Hendey's battle with topical steroid withdrawal.

26. BBC News. (2022, April). *Skin cream withdrawal effects 'need more research'*.

27. HCPLive. (2025). Interview with Dr. Peter Lio at Revolutionizing Atopic Dermatitis (RAD) Conference.

28. Hajar T, Leshem YA, Hanifin JM, Nedorost ST, Lio PA, Paller AS. (2015). A systematic review of topical corticosteroid withdrawal ("steroid addiction") in patients with atopic dermatitis and other dermatoses. *JAAD*, 72(3):541–549. [PubMed 25592622]

29. Juhász MLW, Cohen JM, Mesinkovska NA. (2017). Topical steroid addiction and withdrawal in children: A systematic review. *Pediatric Dermatology*, 34(6):593–601.

30. Sheary B, et al. (2016–2021). Case series and cohort studies on TSW. *Aust Fam Physician* 2016; *Australas J Dermatol* 2018; *Clin Exp Dermatol* 2019; *Dermatitis* 2021.

31. Fukaya M. (2014). Topical steroid addiction in atopic dermatitis. *Drug, Healthcare and Patient Safety*, 6:131–138. [PMC4171913]

32. Silverberg JI, et al. (2024). Patient-reported harm from topical steroids: A multinational survey. *JAAD*; and Ann Allergy Asthma Immunol. (2023). Caregiver survey.

33. Sheary B, et al. (2016–2021). Longitudinal Australian clinic cohorts on TSW. *Aust Fam Physician* 2016; *Australas J Dermatol* 2018; *Clin Exp Dermatol* 2019; *Dermatitis* 2021.

34. UK Medicines and Healthcare products Regulatory Agency (MHRA). (2021). *Topical steroid withdrawal reactions: A review of the evidence.* Gov.uk.

35. World Health Organization (WHO). (2019). *Guidelines for regulatory action on skin-lightening products with steroids and hydroquinone.*

36. Rapaport MJ, Rapaport V. (1999). The red skin syndrome: corticosteroid addiction and withdrawal. *JAAD*, 41(2):311–323; Rapaport MJ, Lebwohl M. (2003). Corticosteroid addiction and withdrawal in the atopic: The red burning skin syndrome. *Clinics in Dermatology*, 21(3):201–214.

37. National Eczema Association. (2020). *Eczema in America Survey.* NEA.org.

38. Pollock BH, Thomas KS, et al. (2021). Harmful skin-lightening products containing corticosteroids: A global public health issue. *British Journal of Dermatology*, 185(6):1087–1095.

39. American Academy of Pediatrics. (2025). Clinical Report on Atopic Dermatitis: Prevalence estimates of 20–25% in children.

40. Tian E, Rauso C, Weidinger S, et al. (2023). Global epide-
miology of atopic dermatitis: A comprehensive systematic
analysis and modelling study. *British Journal of Dermatology*,189(6):659–668.

41. United Nations. (2024). *World Population Prospects 2024*.

CHAPTER SIX

HISTORY OF MIRACLE CREAMS

LET'S GO BACK TO THE BIRTH OF THIS "Miracle Cream." The patterns we've seen across Japan, India, Australia, and the UK aren't just coincidences—they're the natural result of a half-century of medical and marketing history. To understand how millions of people around the world came to rely on a drug capable of causing Topical Steroid Addiction, you have to rewind to the beginning.

The story doesn't start in a dermatology clinic, but in a laboratory—when pharmaceutical companies discovered they could bottle steroids as a "miracle cream," wrap them in promises, and sell them into homes, hospitals, and even baby nurseries. What happened next was not inevitable in nature—it was manufactured.[1, 2, 5]

In 1952, at Columbia-Presbyterian Medical Center in New York, dermatologists Marion B. Sulzberger and Victor H. Witten began applying an experimental compound—hydrocortisone acetate—to inflamed skin. This was not a mass trial, nor a nationwide study. It was, in their own words, a "controlled test" involving just 19 patients suffering from eczema, psoriasis, and other persistent dermatoses.[6] Treatment lasted from several days to a few weeks.

The results were impressive—at least in the short term. Redness faded, swelling went down, and itching subsided. Encouraged, they expanded their investigation. In 1953, they published a follow-up in *JAMA* with 62 patients, now including adults, children, and even infants.[7] Once again, the short-term results were favorable.

What the papers did not report was what happened to these patients months or years later. No one checked for skin thinning under a microscope. No one tested for hypothalamic–pituitary–adrenal (HPA) axis suppression—the measure of whether the drug was affecting adrenal function. No one monitored for rebound flares or dependency.

Yet in the buoyant postwar era, with medicine riding a wave of antibiotic triumphs and vaccine breakthroughs, the absence of bad news was taken as proof of safety.[3] Hydrocortisone was soon hailed as a miracle.

Milestones

- 1952 – Sulzberger & Witten (*Arch Derm Syphilol*): 19 patients, days–weeks treatment, short-term improvement.
- 1953 – Sulzberger & Witten (*JAMA*): 62 patients, including children and infants; no long-term safety data.

The Potency Race

By the late 1950s, drug companies were experimenting with fluorination and other chemical tweaks to make steroids more powerful. The next generation—triamcinolone acetonide, fluocinolone acetonide, and betamethasone valerate—promised stronger, faster suppression of inflammation.[8, 9]

Before launch, these new formulations underwent short-term clinical trials—often just a few weeks—primarily to confirm they reduced visible inflammation faster than hydrocortisone.[1, 3, 10, 9] The testing focused on potency and efficacy, not on long-term safety.[3]

Systemic absorption was sometimes measured using urinary excretion or plasma cortisol suppression, but these were typically single-dose or short-course studies with small numbers of adult subjects.[11, 12, 13] There were no multi-year safety studies, no pediatric safety trials, and no studies during pregnancy for most of these early high-potency agents—and no structured post-marketing surveillance to catch rare or delayed adverse effects.[14]

The same assumption carried over from the early hydrocortisone days: that what was safe short-term in a few dozen people would be safe in broader, long-term use.[5] What wasn't being tracked was the flip side of increased potency: deeper skin penetration, more systemic absorption, and greater risk of both local and whole-body side effects.[14, 9]

Milestone

- Late 1950s–1960s – Introduction of high-potency synthetics: triamcinolone acetonide, fluocinolone acetonide, betamethasone valerate; tested only in short-term trials, no long-term safety data.

The Blanching Test

In 1962, Alexander McKenzie and Robert Stoughton introduced the human vasoconstrictor assay, published in *Archives of Dermatology.*[14] Known as the "blanching test," it involved applying a steroid to the forearm and measuring the degree of skin whitening caused by capillary constriction.

This test became the gold standard for comparing steroid strength. It was quick, reproducible, and ideal for product development—but it had a fatal blind spot. It measured potency, not long-term safety.[3]

Buried in their paper was a warning that should have echoed through every pediatric ward and dermatologist's office:

Occlusion can increase absorption more than 100-fold compared with open application.[14]

That finding meant that covering treated skin—whether with bandages, tight pajamas, or "wet wraps"—could turn a mild cream into a high-dose systemic exposure.[2] But instead of leading to broad public warnings, the data was mostly filed away in specialist circles.

Milestone

- 1962 – McKenzie & Stoughton's blanching assay becomes standard potency test. Key finding: Occlusion boosts absorption more than 100×.

The Consumer Aisle Moment

It was 1979, and the pharmacy aisle had just gotten a new resident. There it sat, between the lip balm and the aspirin—a neat row of small tubes in bright, trustworthy packaging. No white prescription bag. No trip to the doctor. No stern lecture about "only for short-term use." Just a cheerful price sticker and the words *Hydrocortisone 0.25%* printed on the label.[16]

A man wandered in for gum and aspirin, maybe a bottle of shampoo. He spotted the tube—"for itching, rashes, and skin irritation"—and tossed it in his basket without a second thought. Why not? It looked as harmless as toothpaste.[3]

At the checkout counter, there was no warning about keeping it off large areas, no pharmacist asking if he planned to use it on a child, no mention that prolonged use could thin the skin or suppress the adrenal glands.[1] Just the beep of the scanner, a bag with gum, aspirin, and the miracle cream—now available to anyone, for anything, for as long as they felt like using it.

And so hydrocortisone made the quiet leap from prescription drug to casual purchase, its dangers hidden in plain sight, its ability to lead to dependency and higher potency prescriptions unknown.

Milestone

- 1979 – FDA approves OTC hydrocortisone 0.25%, later 0.5% and 1%.

The Addiction Warning

That same year, two dermatologists—Albert Kligman and Peter Frosch—published an article titled "Steroid Addiction."[15] For the first time, the term appeared in the medical literature, describing something chillingly familiar to TSW sufferers: patients whose skin flared worse after stopping long-term steroid use, leading them to restart the cream simply to avoid the rebound.[1]

Kligman and Frosch didn't sugarcoat it:

Finally, what can be done for addicted patients? This is no enterprise for the short-tempered, impatient physician. Withdrawal is agonizing and the doctor must be enrolled in the battle emotionally, providing strenuous support and unremitting encouragement.[15]

Nearly three decades after hydrocortisone's debut, leading dermatologists were openly acknowledging that withdrawal could be severe, prolonged, and emotionally taxing for both patient and physician.[5] Yet their warning never translated into systemic safeguards.

Milestone

- 1979 – Kligman & Frosch publish *Steroid Addiction*; first formal acknowledgment of rebound withdrawal patterns.

Early Cracks in the Miracle

By the 1980s, the sheen on the "miracle cream" had started to dull—not because the drugs stopped working, but because the first real warning signs were appearing in the medical literature.[5]

Doctors began describing perioral dermatitis and steroid-induced rosacea-like eruptions—red, burning, inflamed skin that worsened after the cream was stopped.[1] One case report detailed a man who developed a painful, pustular facial rash after two months of daily high-potency clobetasol 0.05% on his face; it only improved once the steroid was stopped and antibiotics were prescribed.[17] Another review described patients with papules, pustules, swelling, and telangiectasia—tiny, visible blood vessels—as either a direct effect of long-term steroid use or as part of the rebound after stopping.[18]

Skin atrophy—thinning of the skin—also moved from a theoretical risk to a documented reality.[3] Super-potent steroids applied under occlusion could cause visible thinning in as little as a week; even without occlusion, changes were seen in two weeks.[13, 19] The risk climbed with potency, larger application areas, longer use, and, most dramatically, in children.[2]

The systemic effects that early hydrocortisone studies had ignored began showing up, too. FDA data later confirmed that high-potency creams like betamethasone dipropionate suppressed the hypothalamic–pituitary–adrenal (HPA) axis in nearly a third of children aged three months to 12 years after standard use.[20] In adolescents treated with clobetasol lotion for just two weeks, suppression rates climbed to 64%; in adults treated for four weeks, 80%.[20] Even moderate weekly doses—14 grams of clobetasol—could trigger measurable adrenal suppression.[13]

Then came the ocular complications. In one study, seven out of 37 children with eczema developed cataracts after using moderate-potency steroids around their eyes for about six months of each year over five years.[21] These were potent drugs, used off-label on delicate eyelid skin, and the long-term damage was irreversible.[3]

The pattern was consistent across these reports: the more potent the drug, the larger the area treated, the longer the duration, the higher the risk—exactly the scenarios never tested in the original hydrocortisone trials. And yet, despite being documented in the literature, these risks rarely made it into conversations between doctor and patient, much less onto a drug label.[5]

As Potency Ramped Up, So Did TSA

In the early years, during the 1950s and 1960s, few addicted patients were seen because the available steroids were relatively weak. But as the strength of steroids increased, many experts believe the number of addicted patients did also. When prescriptions were lost, not renewed, or therapy stopped, patients developed TSW. In large numbers, doctors attempted to "solve" the problem of red flaring with repeated steroid shots and oral doses. Infections were blamed, hidden allergens were blamed, extensive lab and X-ray tests were ordered, and patients were often admitted to hospitals for IV steroids.[6, 8, 9, 10, 12, 15, 26]

Dates of Steroid Introduction

1950s	1952	Hydrocortisone	Class VII (Least Potent)
	1958	Triamcinoline acetonide	Class IV (Mid-Strength)
1960s	1961	Fluocinolone acetonide	Class VI (Mild)
		Flurandrenolone	Class V (Lower Mid-Strength)
1970s	1971	Desonide	Class V–IV (Lower Mid/Mid-Strength)
		Fluocinonide	Class III–II (Upper Mid-Strength to Potent)
	1974	Clobetasol propionate	Class I (Superpotent)
	1975	Betamethasone dipropionate (as Diprosone™)	Class III–II (Upper Mid-Strength to Potent)
		Desoximetasone	Class II (Potent)
	1976	Hydrocortisone butyrate	Class V (Lower Mid-Strength)
		Diflorasone diacetate	Class I (Superpotent)
	1978	Hydrocortisone valerate	Class IV (Mid-Strength)
1980s	1981	Betamethasone dipropionate (as Diprolene™)	Class II–I (Potent to Superpotent)
	1986	Clobetasol-17-propionate	Class I (Superpotent)
	1989	Alclometasone dipropionate	Class VI (Mild)
1990s	1990	Fluticasone proprionate	Class III (Upper Mid-Strength)
		Mometasone Furoate	Class II (Potent)
	1991	Halobetasol propionate	Class I (Superpotent)

A Lone Voice in Nevada

Not all the early cracks in the miracle cream story came from doctors or journals—some came from the court of law.[5, 1]

In 1997, Leslie Cain Ortega was one of them. A lifelong eczema sufferer, she was prescribed a topical treatment that—unbeknownst to her—contained potent, unlabeled steroids. The result was catastrophic. Leslie developed Cushing's Syndrome, a serious hormonal disorder caused by steroid overexposure.[22, 3]

She didn't just accept her fate. She took Smith Pharmaceuticals to court—and won a $25,000 settlement. Almost thirty years ago, that case set a legal precedent: proof in a courtroom that these drugs could cause lasting harm.[1] The real victory wasn't the money. It was what came next.

Housebound for four years while enduring topical steroid withdrawal syndrome, Leslie turned her personal crisis into public advocacy.[4] She went to the media. Her story appeared in the *Las Vegas Sun*, the *Boston Patriot Ledger*, on local NBC news, and across national radio talk shows.[22, 23]

In 1999, she founded the Steroid Warning Network—the first known patient-led nonprofit devoted to informing and supporting people harmed by steroid-containing medications.[2] That same year, the Nevada State Legislature passed AJR24, a resolution requiring all steroid-containing products sold in the state to be clearly labeled.[24] Leslie's activism was the spark.

The state recognized her organization for its public service. For a moment, it seemed like change was coming. But AJR24 never left Nevada. It carried no real enforcement power—maybe deliberately buried, like other secrets in Nevada's infamous Area 51—and, like so many warnings about these drugs, it was quietly sidelined.[5]

By 2007, the Steroid Warning Network shut its doors, worn down by lack of funding and the burnout of a small, overworked team.[25] Leslie had been a trailblazer—a lone voice in the desert who saw the truth and shouted it into the wind. But the system was louder.

Her story stands as proof: the harm was real, the warnings were there, and the legal precedent was set decades before the world was ready to listen.[1, 3]

Milestone

- 1997 – Landmark court victory and AJR24 steroid-labeling resolution in Nevada; first known patient-led steroid harm nonprofit.

The Legacy of a Half-Story

The history of topical steroids is not just a tale of pharmaceutical innovation—it's a case study in how incomplete science can harden into entrenched practice.[5] The early safety "proof" came from small, short studies in limited patient samples.[6, 7, 1, 3] But once the drugs hit the market, real-world use rapidly outpaced the conditions under which they'd been tested.[2]

That was it. That's all it took for the so-called miracle cream to cross the finish line—a handful of short-term studies, a few decades of unchallenged optimism, and the FDA's stamp of "safe when used as directed."[5] No long-term trials. No tracking for dependency. No public campaign warning of the 100-fold absorption risk.[14, 3]

From the beginning, the data contained warnings—about systemic absorption, about dependency, about the need for emotional and medical support during withdrawal.[13, 14, 15] Those warnings were either ignored or buried, while potencies climbed, product lines multiplied, and global sales soared.[4]

Once the gate was open, the flood came. Big Pharma smelled the money. Dermatologists saw a quick fix—a way to get itchy, desperate patients out of their offices in minutes. Most genuinely believed it was a win-win: clear the rash, send the patient home happy. They didn't know it was a false cure. They didn't see the trapdoor hidden under the relief.[1, 5]

From there, the use of topical steroids didn't just grow—it exploded. More potencies. More formulations. Patients starting younger and using them longer.[2, 4] The miracle cream had gone mass-market, and no one was watching the clock.

This was the miracle cream's true history—half discovery, half denial—and the second half would be written not in glowing journal abstracts, but in the lived experiences of millions of patients.[2]

Today, the reality looks very different.

> # If steroids were discovered today... I don't think they'd receive a licence.[26, 1, 3, 5]
>
> —Dr. George Moncrieff, Past Chair Dermatology Council for England, General Practice and Undergraduate Tutor at Oxford University and The Royal Free Hospital

The line between treatment and harm had always been thinner than anyone wanted to admit. By the time the world realized it, millions had already crossed it.[2]

And yet, for years, these warnings stayed locked in journals and quiet conversations. It wasn't regulators who rang the alarm. It wasn't the companies that made billions selling the creams. The first real resistance came from patients themselves—like Leslie Cain Ortega, myself, and now global patient cries—who learned the hard way that relief had a cost and decided to fight back.[4]

History can feel abstract until it lands in a nursery. The rise of "miracle creams" wasn't just about marketing and medical journals—it was about mothers and fathers rubbing those creams onto fragile infant skin, trusting the experts, believing the labels. What began as a triumph of pharmaceutical science turned into quiet tragedy in family homes across the globe.

The next chapter isn't about molecules or markets. It's about babies who couldn't sleep, toddlers and children who screamed in pain, and parents who were told they were doing everything right—only to watch everything go wrong.

|||||||||||||||||||||||||||||||||||||||||||||||||||||||||||||||||||||||||||||||||||||||||||||||||||||||||||||||||||||||||||||||||||||||||||||||||||||||||||||||||||||||||||||||||||

References

1. Posit #1 — TSW is real.

2. Posit #2 — Prevalence is far higher than admitted.

3. Posit #3 — The harm is real and preventable.

4. Posit #4 — Patterns match globally.

5. Posit #5 — The medical establishment has ignored warning signs for decades.

6. Sulzberger MB, Witten VH. (1952). Effect of topically applied compound F in selected dermatoses. *Archives of Dermatology and Syphilology*, 66(3):323–330.

7. Sulzberger MB, Witten VH. (1953). Use of compound F in dermatologic therapy: A preliminary report. *JAMA*, 152(4):407–412.

8. Kligman AM. (1969). The evolution of topical corticosteroids. *Archives of Dermatology*, 99(6):823–834.

9. Stoughton RB. (1972). The vasoconstrictor assay of topical corticosteroids: New developments. *Archives of Dermatology*, 106(6):773–777.

10. Stoughton RB, McKenzie AW. (1963). Topical corticosteroid absorption and effect: Evaluation by vasoconstrictor assay. *Archives of Dermatology*, 88(1):29–32.

11. McKenzie AW, Atkinson PM. (1964). Topical corticosteroids and systemic absorption measured by urinary excretion. *Archives of Dermatology*, 89(2):199–201.

12. Katz HI, Hien NT, Prawer SE, et al. (1984). Superpotent topical steroids: Effects on the HPA axis and plasma cortisol. *Journal of the American Academy of Dermatology*, 10(3):524–528.

13. Hengge UR, Ruzicka T, Schwartz RA, Cork MJ. (2006). Adverse effects of topical glucocorticosteroids. *Journal of the American Academy of Dermatology*, 54(1):1–15.

14. McKenzie AW, Stoughton RB. (1962). Method for comparing percutaneous absorption of steroids. *Archives of Dermatology*, 86(5):608–610.

15. Kligman AM, Frosch PJ. (1979). Steroid addiction. *Archives of Dermatology*, 115(4):459–460.

16. U.S. Food and Drug Administration (FDA). (1979). Approval of OTC hydrocortisone 0.25%; subsequent approvals for 0.5% and 1%. [Federal Register Notice].

17. Diehl S, Cohen DE. (2021). Topical corticosteroid-induced rosacea-like dermatitis: A case report. *JAAD Case Reports*, 7:623–625.

18. Fisher DA. (2009). Perioral dermatitis and steroid-induced rosacea: Clinical review. *Cutis*, 84(5):251–255.

19. *Steroid-Induced Skin Atrophy.* (2023). Clinical reference summary. U.S. National Institutes of Health / NCBI.

20. U.S. Food and Drug Administration (FDA). (2013). *Label review: Betamethasone dipropionate and clobetasol propionate lotions — HPA axis suppression data.* FDA.gov.

21. Mooney E, Rademaker M. (2015). Ocular complications in children using topical corticosteroids for eczema. *Pediatric Dermatology*, 32(4):476–480.

22. *Las Vegas Sun.* (1999). Coverage of Leslie Cain Ortega's steroid harm case and advocacy.

23. *Boston Patriot Ledger.* (1999). Media coverage of Steroid Warning Network.

24. Nevada State Legislature. (1999). AJR24: Resolution requiring labeling of steroid-containing products.

25. Steroid Warning Network. (2007). Closure announcement.

26. Moncrieff G. (2023). Interview on UK television.

PART III

THE HUMAN TOLL

CHAPTER SEVEN

THE CHILDREN: WHEN FAMILIES ARE DEVASTATED

IIIIIIIIIIIIIIIIIIIIIIIIIIIIIIIIIIIIIIIIIIIIIIIIIIIIIIIIIIIIIIIIIIIIIIIIIIIIIIIIIIIIIIIIIIIIIIIIIIIIIIIIIIIIIIIIIIIIIIIIIIIIIIII

REMEMBER RACHEL—WHO NEARLY LOST her life after a doctor's prescription for steroid cream to treat a tiny patch of eczema landed her in the burn unit—from Chapter 3. Infants and children are the most tragic casualties of this epidemic.[1, 3]

Now close your eyes and come with me. **Imagine the softest, sweetest skin you've ever touched**—creamy, delicate, impossibly smooth. It belongs to a baby, warm against your chest, carrying that unmistakable scent of new life. As your eyes travel from the silk of its skin to the wide, sparkling gaze above it, you see a face lit with joy, innocence, and trust. A tiny human who asks for nothing but protection. Nothing but love.

Let's pause—because here is the unthinkable. Why on earth would anyone coat this most precious treasure in a powerful hormone disruptor? Why would we cover an infant's creamy, perfect skin with an endocrine-altering drug—one never properly tested?[5] Yet that is exactly what happens every single day. To soothe a rash, fragile children are coated in "miracle creams" that seep through their thin skin, infiltrating their bloodstream, altering systems still learning how to function.[2]

The hallmark of topical steroid addiction is a burning sensation. Infants and small children can't put that into words for their parents or doctors. All they can do is scream. And that inability to verbalize pain may be the reason doctors fail to recognize the difference between eczema and steroid withdrawal.[5]

In the next two chapters of the book we turn to the human toll. We'll hear from families devastated by topical steroid withdrawal, and uncover the hidden harms that sit in plain sight—on the skin of children, and in the aisles of your local drug and grocery store.

Here's what can happen when a tube of topical steroids, from the drugstore shelf or a prescription from a doctor's hand, ends up on the fragile skin of a child.

Reader Advisory

The following case studies describe severe suffering in children related to topical steroid use and withdrawal. They may be distressing to read, but they are presented here to illustrate the seriousness of the condition and the urgent need for awareness.

Case Study 1: Isaiah Quinn

We begin with one family's story. Not because it is unique, but because it was one of the first to pull the curtain back on what happens when infants are coated with steroids. It began in 2012, when Isaiah Quinn was only three months old.

The First Signs

Isaiah's parents had no history of eczema in their family. When they brought him to the doctor for what looked like a fingernail scratch on his cheek, they expected reassurance. Instead, they were told it was "eczema." They were told to apply over-the-counter hydrocortisone to his cheek.

The eruption that followed looked nothing like "eczema." His skin turned an angry, spreading red, with sharp demarcation lines around his nose, hands, and feet. His body stopped regulating temperature. He gave off a metallic smell. His kidneys began to fail. His albumin plummeted so low he required transfusions. He was labeled Failure to Thrive.

But every answer from specialists was the same: more steroids, higher potency. When intravenous steroids were given in the hospital, the true nightmare began. His mother said later: "All the suffering up until that moment looked like a cakewalk compared to what followed."[1]

Isaiah's Descent

The first three months of Isaiah's topical steroid withdrawal were, in his mother's words, hell on earth.[1] His only relief came from taking near-constant baths to dull the nerve pain. Sometimes he soaked every two hours around the clock. His parents were sleep-deprived, broken.

Skin-to-skin contact—the most natural comfort between a parent and infant—was impossible. His body radiated unbearable heat. His parents wrapped him in cotton pillowcases to hold him. His mother slept upright in a recliner for eight months, cradling his hands so he wouldn't claw himself bloody in the night.

"Minutes felt like years," she remembered. "There were days I prayed for God to take us all."

The Ripple Effect

The impact on the family was total. Isaiah's father missed work for repeated hospitalizations. His older sister's childhood shrank to hospitals and hushed prayers. Church gatherings, homeschool outings, and family visits all vanished. Their home became a sealed chamber, with detergents, perfumes, even relatives posing danger to Isaiah's raw skin.

"We were stuck in survival mode," his mother said. "Our lives came to a screeching halt."[3]

Encounters with the Medical System

When Isaiah's parents suggested this was not eczema but steroid harm, doctors laughed. One told them to "stop Google diagnosing." Another insisted, "Steroids are the only thing that works."[5]

But one pediatrician listened. He agreed to monitor Isaiah's internals and defend the family against hospital specialists pushing ever-stronger drugs. His quiet advocacy, Isaiah's parents believe, saved not only their son's life but their family from Child Protective Services intervention.[3, 5]

If there is one thing more devastating than watching your child suffer, it is knowing the cause—and being told you are wrong. Parents of children in topical steroid withdrawal live in that twilight zone: certain of what is happening before their eyes, yet dismissed, mocked, or even threatened by the very professionals they turned to for help.[5]

Imagine holding your baby through the night, their skin burning, oozing, and peeling, knowing in your gut that steroids are the problem. And then being told—by the white coat across from you—that you must keep using them or risk losing your child to Child Protective Services (CPS). Finding a sympathetic doctor is paramount to avoid CPS.

Where They Are Now

On May 22, 2013, Isaiah's family stopped all steroids. After going through TSW, his skin is now flawless. Now age 12 he has no memory of the horror.[1] His mother and sister still carry the PTSD, but they also carry gratitude that their story helped light the way for others.

"Would we undo it if we could? Absolutely," his mother says. "But if Isaiah's suffering gave answers to even one family—if his life spared another child this path—then at least the pain was not in vain."[3]

Pain to Power

Isaiah's mother, Stephanie, refused to let her family's suffering be in vain. She took her pain to power by launching a blog that chronicled Isaiah's journey and warned other parents about the dangers of topical steroids. **Over fifteen years of advocacy, she has witnessed hundreds of infants and children go through withdrawal.** Out of that experience, she also created a gift for the community: her handmade nourishing balms, born from the struggle to comfort her own child. Today, her Etsy shop *The Home Herbalist* has nearly 2,000 five-star reviews, a testament to the hope and relief she continues to offer other families walking the same dark road.

Over the years, Stephanie has transformed her family's nightmare into a mission of service, helping hundreds of parents recognize what doctors often dismiss. Her story is not just personal—it is part of a much larger pattern.[4] Because what happened to Isaiah was not an accident, or bad luck. It is the predictable outcome of how children's bodies absorb and respond to these powerful drugs.[3]

The Science of Vulnerability

Children are not just "small adults." Their skin, organs, and immune systems are still developing, which makes them exquisitely vulnerable to the side effects of corticosteroids. When doctors prescribe topical steroids for infants and toddlers, they often do so as if the drug remains on the surface. In reality, a child's skin barrier is thinner and more permeable than an adult's, and systemic absorption is far greater.[1, 3]

That means what is marketed as "just a cream" can act more like an oral or intravenous drug in a baby. Steroids applied even to small areas can slip quickly into the bloodstream, altering hormones, suppressing adrenal glands, and interfering with growth and development.[2, 3]

Researchers have documented the consequences. A 2014 review found:[3]

- HPA axis suppression—stress-response system switched off.
- Iatrogenic Cushing's syndrome—in 35 years, 43 cases documented, 86% in infants.
- Growth retardation, eye damage, bone damage, and even fatal infections.

The review underscored that risk is highest when potent agents are applied to infants, especially over large areas or under occlusion (like diapers). Yet these are the very conditions under which steroids are often prescribed.[5]

Case Study 2: Abby

Abby's mother did what any parent would do when her three-month-old baby developed a rash. She brought her daughter to the doctor. The diagnosis came quickly: eczema. The prescription: topical cortisone, to be applied twice a day until the cheek cleared.

At first, it seemed to work. The small patch faded, only to rebound worse. More trips to the doctor followed, and within two weeks, Abby had been prescribed three different topical steroids. The cycle had begun: brief relief, followed by worse flares, followed by stronger creams. By age two, Abby's "eczema" had spread across her entire body. She scratched until she bled. Sleep vanished for both child and parents.

One desperate night, Abby's mother stumbled onto the ITSAN website. What she read sounded chillingly familiar: sufferers describing dependence on corticosteroids, worsening symptoms over time, and the nightmare of withdrawal. She realized her baby had not just eczema, but steroid addiction.[1]

She stopped the creams immediately. What followed was eighteen months of agony. Abby's skin turned an angry, burning red. Nights were endless with oozing, pain, and screams. Her mother quit her job to care for her very ill child, even as doctors, family, and friends urged her to return to steroids. But she refused. "The risk was too great to turn back," she later said. "I knew they might never work again—and the side effects were too serious to ignore."[3]

Leaning on ITSAN's support group, Abby's mother endured the darkest season of her life. "Had it not been for ITSAN.org, I would have been completely alone in this nightmare," she said. "**This needs to change, and parents like me are not going to stop until something is done about it.**"[4]

Today, Abby is smiling again. The tears, the sleepless nights, and the blood-stained sheets have given way to laughter. Her skin is still recovering, but she has her life back. And her mother has found purpose in sharing their story so no other parent feels as alone as she once did.

The Toll on Families

There is something that may be more terrifying to parents than the actual horror of TSW, and that is losing, or the threat of losing, your child to Child Protective Services. This can be a real outcome when medical dogma and the wrong set of circumstances collide.[5]

Anna was a devoted mother who stopped using topical steroids on her toddler after realizing the creams were making her child's skin worse, not better. When she tried to explain this to her doctors, she was accused of neglect and consulting "Doctor Google." Within days, Child Protective Services was in the picture. The terror of nearly losing custody of her baby—not because she was careless, but because she refused to keep applying the very drug that was harming her child—left scars she still carries today. Her story is not unique. Several families in the TSW community have faced this same nightmare, proving that the damage of topical steroid withdrawal goes far beyond the skin; it shatters trust, security, and the very foundation of family life.[5]

This is just one of the horrors of TSW in children.

Sibling Trauma

Siblings grow up in the shadow of crisis. They watch their baby brother or sister scream through the night, claw their skin raw, soak in endless baths just to survive the pain. They miss school outings, birthday parties, playdates. They learn too young that their parents' attention is consumed by survival, that the sound of laughter has been replaced by the sound of crying. Many carry guilt: Why my sibling and not me? Others carry scars of helplessness that last a lifetime.[2]

Whole Families in Withdrawal

In some households, it isn't just one child who suffers—it is everyone. In the TSW community, there are families where multiple children, and sometimes parents too, were prescribed topical steroids and developed withdrawal at the same time.

One mother of three boys recalled the nightmare of watching each son, at different ages, spiral into steroid addiction under the care of the same dermatologist. "Our home became a haze of skin flakes and endless bath rotations," she said. "Keeping our three boys comfortable was a full-time job."

The family endured together, day after day, **but today all three sons are healed**. Their story is both a testament to resilience—and a chilling warning of how easily entire families can be swept into the cycle.[4]

Marriage Strain

Marriages bend under the relentless weight of TSW. One parent may quit work to become a full-time caregiver, while the other shoulders the financial burden. Sleep deprivation and constant fear leave nerves frayed. Couples who once dreamed together find themselves arguing over treatments, finances, even whether they are strong enough to keep going. Some marriages do not survive. Those that do carry the marks of battle—closer in some ways, shattered in others.[3]

Innocence Lost

TSW robs not just skin, but innocence. The innocence of children, who should be learning to walk, to laugh, to play in the sun—not confined to tubs of water, swaddled in cotton, or hospitalized for drug-induced crises. The innocence of parents, who trusted doctors and the medical system, only to discover that the treatment was the poison. Once you have held a screaming infant whose skin burns from the very drug meant to heal them, you can never go back to blind trust again.[3, 5]

PTSD for the Whole Family

Even after healing, the trauma remains. Parents flinch at the faintest rash, the smell of ointment, the thought of a white coat. Children who recover from TSW often have no memory of their suffering—but their parents do. Night after night of screams that rattled the walls do not vanish. Parents describe the trauma as bone-deep, the kind that reshapes how they see the world forever.

One mother put it plainly: **"We don't just recover from TSW. We survive it. And the survival changes every one of us."**

Former ITSAN president, TSW caregiver and pediatric nurse Kathy Tullos reflected on the deeper tragedy: "It's amazing that when we treated eczema with steroids we caused so much suffering, and when we didn't treat, we returned to simple baseline eczema. I don't think anyone knows what pure eczema looks like anymore."[5]

Case Study 3: Nikki's Daughter

Before we launch into Case Study Three, it's important to say this: we had hundreds of infants and children who could have been included in this chapter. In just one Facebook support group alone—now more than 26,000 members strong—parents have shared stories of their babies suffering through topical steroid withdrawal. We chose these three cases not to shield the truth, but to prevent this chapter from becoming unbearable in its repetition of horror.[2]

Nikki, a young mother, was told by her doctor that topical steroids were "perfectly safe" for babies. She used the cream on her infant daughter's cheek for only one week. That was all it took. When she stopped, her baby's skin exploded with oozing, crusting, itching, and swelling—one hundred times worse than the eczema that had started it all. Furious and heartbroken, Nikki did the only thing she could think of: she posted her baby's photos online with her story, determined to warn other parents before they made the same mistake.[1, 3]

The images of Nikki's baby are almost unbearable to look at. Her tiny body in a onesie, skin caked in scabs and cracked open, her eyes swollen nearly shut—all from only one week of steroid use. It is grotesque and searing, the kind of image you can never unsee. And yet, in the TSW community, photos like this are posted daily by desperate parents begging to be believed.[1] When I've felt exhausted writing this book, or worn down from years in the TSW fight, I sometimes pull out those pictures. They remind me exactly why I cannot stop. Why none of us can.[4]

One of Many TSW Toddlers

It's important to note that Nikki is not alone. Many mothers, desperate to be believed, have turned to Instagram to document their toddlers' suffering. One such mom is known online as @ToddlerTSW. Her account has become one of the most visible examples of what this epidemic looks like in children, with over 16,000 followers. We'll learn her story in more detail in the upcoming Social Media Revolution chapter, but her presence online is already a powerful reminder: parents are no longer suffering in silence—they are reaching out to the world for help.[4]

The suffering of these children is a warning sign. It shows us not only how vulnerable babies are to steroid addiction, but also how invisible the danger has become. Families think they are reaching for comfort, not realizing that the very creams lining baby aisles can be the start of the nightmare.[1, 3]

Right now, in drugstores across America, parents can find *Aquaphor Itch Relief Cream* stocked in the baby department. Its label doesn't scream danger, sometimes it even carries pictures of a cartoon character or a butterfly—but inside the tube is 1% hydrocortisone, a steroid strong enough to start the cycle of dependence.[3, 5]

And it is far from the only hidden harm out there—not just for babies, but for us all.[2]

References

1. Posit #1 — TSW is real.

2. Posit #2 — Prevalence is far higher than admitted.

3. Posit #3 — The harm is real and preventable.

4. Posit #4 — Patterns match globally.

5. Posit #5 — The medical establishment has ignored warning signs for decades.

6. Hengge UR, Ruzicka T, Schwartz RA, Cork MJ. (2006). Adverse effects of topical glucocorticosteroids. *Journal of the American Academy of Dermatology*, 54(1):1–15.

7. Tempark T, Phatarakijnirund V, Chatproedprai S, et al. (2014). Systemic side-effects of topical corticosteroids in children. *Pediatric Dermatology*, 31(6):619–624.

CHAPTER EIGHT

HIDDEN HARM: HOW TO PROTECT YOURSELF AND YOUR FAMILY

||||||||||||||||||||||||||||||||||||||||||||||||||||||||||||||||||||||||||||||||||||||||||||||||||||||||||||||||||||||||||||||||||||||

IT'S ONE THING TO READ A LABEL AND know you're taking a medication—prescription or over-the-counter, spelled out plainly on the package. At least then you know what you're dealing with. But what if those same steroids were hiding in products that whisper safety—"natural," "gentle," "PABA-free"? What if they were buried inside creams and cosmetics—the lotion by your sink, the soothing ointment in your nightstand, the makeup you use every day?[2]

That's when the nightmare doesn't announce itself. It slips quietly into your life, in disguise.

And it isn't just baby creams or "botanical" moisturizers. Hemorrhoid ointments and feminine itch creams—staples in American bathrooms—often contain topical steroids strong enough to trigger dependency. **Because they're sold as comfort products, most users never realize they're medicating their skin** with the very same class of drugs linked to withdrawal and damage.[3] Add to that the cosmetics aisle, where "fade" creams, makeup, and even luxury lotions have been caught hiding undisclosed corticosteroids, and the problem becomes systemic.[5]

A Jar on the Counter

Picture this: A woman in her 30s finally treats herself to a little indulgence. The white Mario Badescu jar with green lettering sits on her bathroom counter—its branding promising botanical healing. At around $25 for a two-ounce jar, it feels like a modest luxury—not drugstore cheap, not designer expensive. Each morning, before work, she smooths it over her cheeks and forehead. The texture is silky, the scent delicate. She looks in the mirror and believes she's investing in confidence, in being more polished, more herself.

At first, it seems to work. Her skin looks calmer, more even, a little glowier. She tells friends she's struck gold. The jar becomes part of her identity—a quiet magic she carries into her day.

Then the promise sours. The smooth cover gives way to a subtle sting, and then a red flush. The flush morphs into burning, then itching. When the rash blooms across her face, she can't stand to look at herself anymore.[1]

Down the rabbit hole she goes—dermatologist after dermatologist, each offering something stronger: steroid creams, thicker ointments, pills to calm the inflammation. Relief is temporary. Relapse is relentless. She slips into a cycle she never wanted.[3]

What she didn't know—what the jar's soft green label didn't tell her—was that the "botanical" cream was secretly harboring potent steroids. The drug she thought she dodged was in the product she trusted most.[5]

Not Alone

This woman was not alone. In fact, she became part of a class-action lawsuit against Mario Badescu.

In 2013, two of the brand's most popular creams—Control Cream and Healing Cream—were revealed to contain unlabeled corticosteroids (hydrocortisone and triamcinolone acetonide). Neither appeared on the ingredient lists. The products were marketed as "gentle" and "botanical," but in reality they carried drugs potent enough to cause skin thinning, redness, burning, and dependency.[1, 3] After regulators overseas tested the products and confirmed the steroids, lawsuits followed in the United States. Plaintiffs alleged that thousands of unsuspecting customers had been exposed to hidden steroids, many suffering skin damage as a result.

The *definitive expert* on topical steroid addiction and withdrawal was sought out by the attorneys who filed a class action suit against Mario Badescu; they flew **Marvin J. Rapaport to Washington D.C. and hired him as their expert**.

Mario Badescu eventually settled the case, offering restitution to affected customers—but without admitting wrongdoing. Regulatory agencies, including the Korean Ministry of Food and Drug Safety, had already suspended sales after detecting the unlabeled steroids, adding international weight to the claims.[5]

A Pattern of Deception

Mario Badescu was not an isolated incident.

- **Skin-Cap (Cheminova, 1997):** Marketed as an over-the-counter zinc spray for eczema, Skin-Cap was pulled from shelves after FDA testing found undisclosed clobetasol propionate—one of the most potent topical steroids available.[3] Class certification was upheld by the Alabama Supreme Court, with the core issue being undisclosed steroids.[5]

- **Beauty Supply Fade Creams:** A 2024 dermatology investigation found prescription-strength corticosteroids, including clobetasol and betamethasone, in "fade" creams sold openly in beauty supply stores in U.S. cities such as Miami, Washington D.C., and Baltimore. These products, marketed as cosmetic skin lighteners, often target women of color—a public health time bomb hiding in plain sight.[2, 3]

- **International Skin-Lightening Creams:** Health Canada and the FDA continue to seize imported cosmetics found to contain hidden steroids, sometimes in combination with hydroquinone and mercury. Academic reviews confirm dozens of such seizures globally, with corticosteroids being the most common undisclosed active.[2, 5]

Protecting Your Family

Hidden steroids don't just appear in exotic imported creams or mis-labeled luxury products. They show up in the everyday items people buy and use without a second thought. Here are the categories where risk has been documented:

- **Poison ivy and anti-itch treatments** — many contain hydrocortisone 1% as the active ingredient (e.g., Cortizone-10 Anti-Itch, Aveeno 1% Hydrocortisone Anti-Itch Cream).[3]
- **Baby rash relief creams** — some "gentle" rash ointments have been found with hidden steroids, especially imported brands seized by regulators. Even *Aquaphor Itch Relief Cream*, sold in the baby aisle, contains hydrocortisone 1%.[2, 3]
- **Baby itch creams** — OTC "eczema relief" creams for infants sometimes feature steroids without parents realizing it.[2]
- **Cosmetic "control" creams and makeup primers** — Mario Badescu's "Control Cream" and "Healing Cream" contained unlabeled hydrocortisone and triamcinolone acetonide, leading to lawsuits.[1, 3, 5]
- **Redness-relief skincare** — creams marketed for rosacea or redness (often labeled "calming" or "botanical") have been flagged overseas for hiding steroids like clobetasol.[2]
- **Vaginal itch creams** — products like *Vagisil Anti-Itch Cream* or *Monistat Itch Relief* often include hydrocortisone as the active agent.[3]

- **Hemorrhoid creams and ointments** — common bathroom-cabinet products like *Preparation H Hydrocortisone 1%* contain topical steroids strong enough to trigger dependency if overused.[3]
- **Skin-lightening and "fade" creams** — beauty supply store products marketed for pigmentation and lightening have been repeatedly found to contain potent undisclosed steroids (clobetasol, betamethasone).[2, 3, 5, 10]
- **Imported cosmetics** — lotions, ointments, and "herbal" creams from Asia, Africa, and Latin America are frequently seized by FDA and Health Canada for hidden steroids (sometimes alongside mercury and hydroquinone).[2, 5]
- **Eczema "flare control" lotions** — mainstream OTC brands sometimes sell "eczema control" products with 1% hydrocortisone, often marketed as "gentle" without emphasizing that it's a steroid.[3]
- **Insect bite ointments and first-aid creams** — hydrocortisone-based formulas are a staple in U.S. first-aid kits, often overlooked because they're bundled as simple "anti-itch" creams.[3]
- **Lip Balms** — some lip balms also contain steroids. One such product is *Lovely Skin Fix My Skin Healing Lip Balm* with 1% hydrocortisone.[12]

The Takeaway

The cases speak for themselves: botanical creams that weren't botanical. Cosmetic fade creams that hid prescription drugs. Soothing ointments that caused burning dependency.[1]

Families cannot assume that a product's branding, price point, or placement on the store shelf makes it safe. Whether it's the baby aisle, the bathroom cabinet, or the makeup bag, the risk is the same: powerful steroids, hidden in plain sight.[3]

And as alarming as that is, these hidden dangers are only part of the story. Because the problem doesn't stop at creams, lotions, or cosmetics. The reach of steroids extends far beyond the skin—into pills, injections, and systemic treatments that carry their own hidden costs.[5]

That's where we go next. The first step in protecting your family is awareness: read every label, question "gentle" claims, and remember that if a product soothes by altering the skin, it may carry hidden risks.

IIIIIIIIIIIIIIIIIIIIIIIIIIIIIIIIIIIIIIIIIIIIIIIIIIIIIIIIIIIIIIIIIIIIIIIIIIIIIIIIIIIIIIIIIIIIIIIIIIIIIIIIIIIIIIIIIIIIIIIIIIIIIIIIIIIIIIIIIIIIIIIIIIIIIIIIIIIIIII

References

1. Posit #1 — TSW is real.

2. Posit #2 — Prevalence is far higher than admitted.

3. Posit #3 — The harm is real and preventable.

4. Posit #4 — Patterns match globally.

5. Posit #5 — The medical establishment has ignored warning signs for decades.

6. Restaino v. Mario Badescu Skin Care, Inc. (2013). Class Action Complaint. Plaintiffs alleged Control Cream and Healing Cream contained undisclosed hydrocortisone and triamcinolone acetonide. Whitfield Bryson & Mason LLP served as plaintiffs' counsel.

7. Korean Ministry of Food and Drug Safety. (2013). Regulatory notice suspending sales of Mario Badescu products after detecting undisclosed corticosteroids.

8. Cheminova America Corp. v. Corker, 726 So. 2d 1237 (Ala. 1999). Alabama Supreme Court affirming class certification in Skin-Cap case involving undisclosed clobetasol.

9. U.S. Food and Drug Administration (1997, 2024). Warning letters and advisories on Skin-Cap aerosol spray containing undisclosed corticosteroids.

10. Campbell J, Perez M, Woolery-Lloyd H. (2024). *Hidden topical corticosteroids in cosmetic fade creams sold in the U.S. Journal of Drugs in Dermatology,* 23(6).

11. Health Canada. (2022). Enforcement notifications and seizures of unauthorized cosmetics containing undisclosed corticosteroids. See also: *Cosmetics Regulatory Journal,* 2022.

12. Fix My Skin website (2025)

CHAPTER NINE

BEYOND SKIN STEROIDS

SHE'S A YOUNG MOM WITH ECZEMA. Every night before bed, she smooths a thin layer of topical steroid cream on the red patches inside her elbows and the back of her hands. It keeps the night time itching away—the doctor called it safe, even gentle.[1]

In the mornings, she reaches for a familiar bottle of Flonase. Allergies run her down every spring, and the spray clears her sinuses enough to pack lunches and get her kids to school. In her purse sits an asthma inhaler—another steroid, taken in quick puffs whenever her chest feels tight. Postpartum, she kept a tube of hemorrhoid ointment by the bathroom sink, just one more cream in the daily rotation. And after a bout of LASIK irritation, she added hydrocortisone eye drops to the mix.

Each product came from a different doctor, a different aisle, a different part of life. None of them asked what else she was using. Each prescription or over-the-counter remedy felt small, isolated, harmless on its own.[2]

But her adrenal glands don't see it that way. They don't know the difference between a cream, a spray, a puff, or a drop.

The adrenal gland doesn't care where it comes from. It just knows: steroids are steroids.[3]

All Steroids Add Up

The body does not distinguish between a steroid applied to the skin, inhaled into the lungs, sprayed into the nose, dripped into the eye, or absorbed rectally. To the hypothalamic-pituitary-adrenal (HPA) axis, every route is cumulative. Each milligram adds to the same internal burden.

Allergy and immunology research confirms this. Clinical reviews warn that intranasal and inhaled corticosteroids, when used together, have additive effects on adrenal suppression.[6, 7, 8, 9] In other words, the risks do not simply overlap—they stack. The more routes of exposure, the greater the chance of systemic complications.

Endocrinology guidelines extend this principle across all routes: oral, inhaled, nasal, topical, ocular, rectal, and injected. The Society for Endocrinology in the UK has gone so far as to recommend Steroid Emergency Cards for patients at risk, emphasizing that multiple small exposures can combine into a dangerous total dose.[12]

And yet, stewardship remains uneven. In asthma care, the allergy and immunology community has begun developing formal frameworks for oral corticosteroid stewardship, focusing on limiting lifetime exposure.[13] But in dermatology, there is none. No system to track cumulative steroid use. No alerts when patients stack prescriptions from different specialties. No counseling to account for hidden over-the-counter creams. Skin patients, perhaps more than any others, are at risk of unknowingly piling steroids from multiple sources, while every gland in their body keeps the true tally.[5]

The Billion-Dollar Business

If you want to understand why stewardship lags, follow the money.[5]

Picture a sleek glass boardroom at GSK's London headquarters. The quarterly earnings call is underway. Slides flash across a projector screen: Trelegy Ellipta, $3.46 billion in sales for 2024.[25] Executives smile, analysts nod, and the number gets circled in red ink as proof of another strong year. For one inhaler brand, that's more than most nonprofits will ever see in a lifetime.

At AstraZeneca, the story is much the same. Symbicort pulled in $2.9 billion last year, and its sibling Breztri added nearly a billion more.[26] With just three inhalers, over $7 billion dollars flowed through corporate pipelines in twelve months.

Step back and the picture grows even bigger. Globally, the corticosteroid market is valued at $5 to $6 billion a year and climbing steadily.[27] Inhaled and nasal steroids dominate the charts. Ophthalmic drops add another $1.5 billion. Analysts peg topical corticosteroids as high as $8 billion, depending on how they're counted.[28] The numbers don't always line up neatly, but that's the point—the money is so vast and so fragmented that even the bean counters can't agree.

And then there's the consumer layer—where steroids are sold as "wellness." OTC brands like Flonase nasal spray and Preparation H hydrocortisone cream sit comfortably inside Haleon's £11.2 billion empire, with Respiratory Health alone accounting for 15 percent of revenue.[29] **These aren't marketed like drugs. They're marketed like lifestyle products.** Hidden steroids, sold with the same cheery language as vitamins and toothpaste.

Billions flow through corporate pipelines every year. And every dollar is tied to someone's adrenal gland, someone's bones, someone's skin.[3]

Systemic Treatments—The Overload

Dermatologists don't just write prescriptions for topical steroid creams. It is common practice to give steroid pills and injections— even for something as routine as eczema. While this book focuses on topical steroid addiction and withdrawal, the reality is that systemic corticosteroids are often handed out for skin problems as well. And when patients already face hidden steroid exposure from creams, sprays, and drops, adding oral or injectable steroids only compounds the damage.[3, 6, 7, 8, 13]

Steroids don't stop at the skin. They seep into nearly every corner of medicine—and every form carries its own hidden cost. It's way beyond just skin.

- **Oral steroids (Prednisone, etc.)** — the "miracle pill" that gives energy and relief, then leaves patients with bone loss, mood swings, and adrenal collapse.[6, 7, 16]
- **Injectables (Kenalog, Depo-Medrol)** — the cortisone shot that quiets pain for a season but chips away at long-term adrenal health.[6, 7, 16]
- **Inhalers** — the billion-dollar backbone of asthma and COPD care, delivering daily doses of hidden dependency.[20, 21]
- **Nasal sprays** — sold over the counter, used for years by allergy sufferers who never realize they're taking a corticosteroid every morning.[9, 10]
- **Eye drops** — a tiny drop that feels local, but up to 80% slips into the bloodstream, adding silently to the body's total load.[14, 15, 17]
- **Topical creams** — the familiar "miracle creams," but now understood as part of a much larger web of exposure.[1, 6, 24]

Stewardship (Where It Exists—and Where It Doesn't)

In medicine, when drugs are potent and pervasive, stewardship becomes a moral imperative. That's why allergy, immunology, and respiratory specialists are pioneering steroid stewardship—a structured, rational approach that balances benefit and risk through education, dosing oversight, and monitoring systems.[13] Patient advocates such as the Global Allergy & Asthma Patient Platform have rallied for it, particularly to minimize repeated lifetime exposure to powerful oral steroids and protect against long-term harm.[12]

Endocrinologists have gone further still: in the United Kingdom, the Society for Endocrinology recommends Steroid Emergency Cards for patients exposed to multiple routes—it's a clear acknowledgment that steroid exposure is cumulative.[11]

Yet in dermatology, where eczema patients are often the most exposed to overlapping steroid sources, stewardship is effectively nonexistent.[5] Every dermatologist knows that steroids applied to broken or inflamed skin enter the bloodstream—but few systems exist to track how much that adds to inhalers, eye drops, nasal sprays, or oral bursts.[6, 7, 24] This is not just an oversight—it's a gap we can no longer afford to ignore.[3, 5]

The Human Toll

Behind every billion-dollar sales figure is a family, a household, a body carrying the weight of steroids.[1] These drugs are not confined to rare diseases or hospital wards—they're in the medicine cabinets of ordinary homes everywhere. A dad with seasonal allergies sprays his nose every morning before work.[9] A teen athlete gets a cortisone shot to stay in the game.[6] A mom keeps a tube of hydrocortisone cream for poison ivy in the summer.[3] A grandmother uses steroid eye drops after cataract surgery.[14]

Each product is prescribed or purchased in isolation, often without a second thought. But taken together, they form a picture of a population quietly medicating itself with some of the most powerful drugs modern medicine has ever created. **This is not fringe. This is everyday life.**[2]

And now imagine those same families where someone is also prescribed topical steroids, tube after tube after tube by a dermatologist—layered on top of the sprays, pills, shots, and drops already in play. The cumulative load becomes staggering, yet it is rarely acknowledged.[5]

The toll is rarely obvious at first. Fatigue that lingers. Bones that weaken sooner than they should. Blood sugar creeping upward. Mood swings that strain relationships. A sense of dependence on products that promise comfort but quietly reshape the body's chemistry.[3]

And yet, the marketing tells another story: comfort, relief, wellness. Steroids are packaged in pastel tubes and cheerful sprays, sold with the same ease as toothpaste or vitamins.[29] They look harmless, but the body keeps score.[5]

This is the paradox at the heart of steroids "beyond skin." They are everywhere—inhaled, sprayed, swallowed, injected, dripped into the eye—woven into daily routines so seamlessly that most people never stop to ask: What is all this adding up to?[2]

The answer is sobering. Cushing's syndrome. Glaucoma. Cataracts. Osteoporosis and brittle bones. Avascular necrosis of the hip. Suppressed adrenal glands. Stunted growth in children. Weight gain, diabetes, and high blood pressure. Mood swings, depression, even psychosis. Increased risk of infection. Thinning skin that tears easily, slow wound healing, and stretch marks etched deep into the body.[6, 7, 8, 11, 12, 13, 16, 17] And what this book is about: Topical Steroid Addiction and Topical Steroid Withdrawal Syndrome.[1]

We've seen the toll—on children, on families, in drugstore aisles, and in every hidden route steroids take into our bodies. We've counted the costs, from broken bones to broken trust, from cataracts to Cushing's, from fatigue to full-blown dependency. And when the human toll is this vast, it is no wonder there is addicted skin around the globe.[2] What began as isolated suffering soon revealed itself as a worldwide crisis—one too loud, too visible, and too devastating to be dismissed. The next three chapters trace how raw pain transformed into collective fire: from the first voices crying out across continents, to the birth of an organized movement, to the social media wave that carried our message farther than we ever imagined. This is where the fight ignites.[4, 5]

‖‖‖

References

1. Posit #1 — TSW is real.

2. Posit #2 — Prevalence is far higher than admitted.

3. Posit #3 — The harm is real and preventable.

4. Posit #4 — Patterns match globally.

5. Posit #5 — The medical establishment has ignored warning signs for decades.

6. Hengge UR, Ruzicka T, Schwartz RA, Cork MJ. Adverse effects of topical glucocorticosteroids. *J Am Acad Dermatol.* 2006;54(1):1–15. Comprehensive review of local and systemic side effects including HPA axis suppression, skin atrophy, ocular complications, osteoporosis, and infection risk.

7. Dhar S, Seth J, Parikh D. Systemic Side-Effects of Topical Corticosteroids. *Indian J Dermatol.* 2014;59(5):460–465. Summarizes percutaneous absorption and systemic harms including growth suppression, Cushing's syndrome, and HPA suppression.

8. DiRuggiero D, DiRuggiero M. The Systemic Impact of Topical Corticosteroids in Dermatology. *J Clin Aesthet Dermatol.* 2025;18(1–2 Suppl 1):S16–S20. Discusses the broader systemic burden of topical corticosteroids and calls for stewardship across specialties.

9. Allen DB. Systemic effects of intranasal steroids: an endocrinologist's perspective. *J Allergy Clin Immunol.* 2000;106(4):S179–S190. Documents systemic absorption of intranasal corticosteroids and additive risk when combined with inhaled steroids.

10. Sowerby LJ, Fowler J. Systemic absorption of intranasal corticosteroids may have systemic effects and can add to overall corticosteroid load. *CMAJ.* 2014;186(16):1241–1245. Warns about cumulative systemic risk of intranasal + inhaled corticosteroids.

11. Society for Endocrinology (UK). *Exogenous steroids in adults – adrenal insufficiency guidance.* 2021. Advises that all steroid routes (oral, inhaled, nasal, topical, ocular, rectal, injected) are cumulative; recommends Steroid Emergency Cards for high-risk patients.

12. Global Allergy & Asthma Patient Platform (GAAPP). *Steroid Stewardship Initiative.* 2023. Patient advocacy resource emphasizing cumulative dose awareness, education, and limiting lifetime exposure.

13. Besemer F, et al. Adrenal insufficiency in corticosteroid use: a systematic review. *Lancet Diabetes Endocrinol.* 2021;9(12):863–872. Meta-analysis confirming HPA suppression risk across inhaled and nasal corticosteroids.

14. Medsafe NZ. A drop in the eye has widespread ripples. *Prescriber Update.* Dec 2019. Notes that only 5–10% of an eye drop remains ocular, with up to 80% absorbed systemically.

15. Farkouh A, et al. Systemic side effects of eye drops: a pharmacokinetic perspective. *Clin Ophthalmol.* 2016;10:2433–2441. Details systemic absorption of ophthalmic corticosteroids and potential systemic adverse effects.

16. Schäcke H, Döcke WD, Asadullah K. Mechanisms involved in the side effects of glucocorticoids. *Pharmacol Ther.* 2002;96(1):23–43. Summarizes mechanisms behind systemic harms: osteoporosis, diabetes, hypertension, mood changes, psychiatric effects.

17. National Eye Institute. *Corticosteroids and Eye Health.* NEI Fact Sheet, 2022. Identifies glaucoma and cataracts as key risks from steroid use.

18. Campbell J, Perez M, Woolery-Lloyd H. Hidden Topical Corticosteroids in Cosmetic Fade Creams Sold in the U.S. *J Drugs Dermatol.* 2024;23(6). Documents undisclosed steroids in U.S. beauty-supply creams.

19. Restaino v. Mario Badescu Skin Care, Inc. Class Action Complaint, 2013. Plaintiffs alleged Mario Badescu's Control Cream and Healing Cream contained undisclosed hydrocortisone and triamcinolone.

20. Korean Ministry of Food and Drug Safety. *Suspension of Mario Badescu creams containing undisclosed steroids.* Regulatory Notice, 2013.

21. Cheminova America Corp. v. Corker, 726 So. 2d 1237 (Ala. 1999). Class certification upheld in Skin-Cap litigation; FDA had identified undisclosed clobetasol propionate in "zinc" creams/sprays.

22. U.S. Food and Drug Administration. *Warning: Skin-Cap aerosol spray may contain undisclosed corticosteroids.* FDA Advisory, Oct 2024.

23. Health Canada. *Summary of Enforcement Notifications: Cosmetic and Skin-Lightening Products.* 2022. Lists seizures of imported creams containing clobetasol, betamethasone, hydroquinone, and mercury.

24. Hengge UR, et al. Topical glucocorticoids and systemic side effects. *Curr Opin Investig Drugs.* 2000;1(3):301–309. Notes systemic harms from cumulative percutaneous absorption.

25. GSK plc. *Annual Report 2024.* Reports Trelegy Ellipta net sales of $3.46B.

26. AstraZeneca plc. *Annual Report 2024.* Reports Symbicort ~$2.9B and Breztri ~$978M in revenue.

27. Market Research Future. *Global Corticosteroids Market Report 2024.* Estimates market size at ~$5.2B in 2023, CAGR 7.5%.

28. GlobalData Healthcare. *Topical Corticosteroids Market Analysis.* 2024. Estimates topical steroid market ~$8.4B globally.

29. Haleon plc. *Annual Report 2024.* Consumer Health revenue £11.2B; Respiratory Health 15% of revenue (includes Flonase).

PART IV

THE FIGHT IGNITES

CHAPTER TEN

ADDICTED SKIN AROUND THE WORLD

||||||||||||||||||||||||||||||||||||||||||||||||||||||||||||||||||||||||||||||||||||||||||||||||||||||||||||||||||||||||||||||||||||||||||||||

FROM THE EARLIEST TSW VOICES CRYING out across continents, to the birth of an organized movement, to the social media wave that carried our message far beyond what we imagined—this is where the fight began to burn.

For me, it started with a single night that changed everything. I was about to drop a pebble in a pond that—fifteen years later—has swelled into a tsunami.

Let's pick up here from the end of the earlier *Down the Rabbit Hole* chapter, where I had finished telling my personal TSA story—the night I discovered the truth. In a nod to one of my favorite and iconic sci-fi movies from 1999, *The Matrix*, let's just say I followed the white rabbit. **Only in my story, the white rabbit had a name: Dr. Rapaport.**

The glow of my computer screen had barely faded from that night—the night Dr. Marvin Rapaport's words pulled me back from the edge. *You are not crazy. You are not alone. You can heal.*

When you've been drowning for years, and someone throws you a lifeline, you don't just grab it—you hold on with everything you have. And once you're safe enough to breathe, you start looking around for others who are still sinking.

I was so overjoyed to finally have the answer—*my answer*—that I couldn't keep it to myself. The truth I'd clawed out of the dark at 12:30 a.m. couldn't stay hidden in the fine print of a medical journal. I had to drag it into the light. I had to put it where any desperate soul, anywhere in the world, could find it.

So, with my skin raw and my red burning hands, I opened my laptop again. This time, not to search for a cure—but to build a beacon.

So I built that beacon—even as my own skin burned, peeled, and wept. While I was going through Topical Steroid Withdrawal Syndrome (TSW) myself, I was also trying to send up a flare for others lost in the dark.

TSW comes after one's skin becomes addicted to steroids—when you stop the steroids causing the addiction. It is, for most people, like walking through hell. You've already read about the depths of my own suffering in the addiction phase, so I'll say this much here: the years I spent in full-body eczema, and my skin getting prescribed steroid after steroid, were a cakewalk compared to what TSW put me through. And I'm a breast cancer survivor—that was easy by comparison.

Warriors to Advocates

TSW is traumatic. Life-stopping. Soul-shaking. And yes—at times, it brought me to the brink. I wondered if I could go on, and didn't care if I lived or died. That feeling isn't unique to me. It's a common sentiment among TSW sufferers—or "warriors," as many of us now call ourselves.

You've heard some of the children's stories in Chapter 7, and you'll hear more later in this book. Through these stories, you'll see the unbearable symptoms and the all-too-common emotional collapse. For now, I'll spare you the graphic details of my own descent—because, to be honest, I can only revisit so much of it without triggering what the community calls TSW PTSD.

That's right—seven little letters that sound like alphabet soup but carry the weight of a thousand sleepless nights and untold painful symptoms.

In a Nutshell: What is TSA/TSW?

Think of topical steroid addiction (TSA) and withdrawal (TSW) as your skin getting hooked on a drug. At first, steroid creams squeeze blood vessels shut and calm the redness—a miracle! But over time, your skin adapts, craving a stronger anti-inflammatory effect and more frequent doses. The barrier gets weaker, the immune system gets tricked, and your skin's "volume knob" for inflammation keeps getting turned up. When you finally stop, the rebound is brutal: blood vessels swing wide open, nitric oxide floods back,[2] and your skin burns, oozes, and flares far worse than the original rash. The most common telltale signs are the burning and the fact that skin turns very red, which is why another popular term for TSA is *Red Skin Syndrome*.[1] In short: steroids don't just stop working—they create a cycle of dependence and withdrawal that looks nothing like normal eczema.

And here's the other layer people don't talk about: these creams are way more than "skin deep." They are body-altering hormones. Steroids can seep in, tinker with your HPA axis (the body's stress-hormone control center), and ripple through the endocrine system.[3, 4] What does that mean long-term? Honestly, no one fully knows—because the medical establishment has never truly acknowledged TSA/TSW, much less funded proper research.[5] So patients are left living out the experiment that science has refused to run.

The Good News/The Bad News

The Good News: Most people who make it through withdrawal fully recover—and many say their skin ends up healthier, stronger, and more resilient than at any point in their lives. My own example is my childhood hand eczema, which turned into decades of adult hand eczema where I consistently used steroid creams as prescribed. After years of "hamburger-meat" hands during TSW, my hands are now creamy, smooth, and completely free of a lifetime of eczema. Anecdotal, yes—but I believe my steroid creams perpetuated my decades of eczema.

The Bad News: Getting there can feel like a nightmare. Withdrawal often takes two to five years on average.[6] Note: that's an average—I myself took over ten years to fully heal. There is even a long-hauler group on Facebook with members well past the averages. On a more upbeat note, some people recover in under a year. Again, no formal research on this, but experts believe recovery time is linked to factors such as length of usage, potency of the steroid, and route of use (topical creams, oral steroids, or injections)[7]—and the overall steroid load we talked about in the last chapter.

You've heard the symptoms: burning, red skin, oozing, flaking, body-temperature swings, hair loss, elephant skin, sleepless nights, and the horrific itch that tests every ounce of patience and resilience one has.[8] Unraveling mental health. The most poignant description I've ever heard of TSW was a poem created by the TSW community in Chapter 16, entitled *Why We Fight.*

Skin is the body's largest organ—our interface with the world, our boundary, and our protection. When TSW takes over, it doesn't just touch a patch here or there; it consumes the entire surface area of that organ and disrupts many systems in the body. **To dismiss or minimize it as "just a skin condition" or "worsening eczema" is dehumanizing.** For me, ten years of TSW was a sentence—a painful prison that held me captive in my own body.

What kept me going through those pitch-black days was purpose. The moment I shifted my focus from my own pain to helping others, something cracked open. I had to believe there was meaning in my suffering—and I found that meaning in Dr. Marvin Rapaport's work. His clinical paper didn't just save me; it lit a fire in me. I knew I couldn't let this truth stay hidden in the pages of a medical journal. So I built a platform to share it.

While my skin peeled and itched and I survived on 15-minute increments of sleep, I launched a website in 2009: AddictedSkin.org.

It wasn't fancy. It was raw and simple—just like me at the time. The site told my story: how doctors took a case of mild eczema and, with good intentions and bad medicine, spiraled it into a full-body health crisis. But more importantly, it highlighted Dr. Rapaport's groundbreaking paper, *Eyelid Dermatitis to Red Skin Syndrome to Cure.* I wanted the world to see what I saw—the truth behind the suffering.

Dr. Rapaport was brilliant, compassionate, and brave. But he wasn't an internet guy. He had no online presence, no public-facing content, no videos or blogs. He was too busy actually saving lives in his clinic to promote his work. But I had digital skills—and fire in my belly.

Back in 2009, the internet wasn't what it is today. YouTube was still in its infancy—clunky, uncurated, just starting to grow. (In 2012, it had fewer than a billion users; by 2025, that number would triple.) There wasn't a single blog, video, or even a comment thread that mentioned Red Skin Syndrome or Topical Steroid Withdrawal Syndrome. No hashtags. No Reddit Rowdies. Just silence.

The only reason I even found Dr. Rapaport's paper was because I used my old pharmaceutical sales chops to dig through PubMed like a research bloodhound. I eventually located the life-saving article—and paid $70 to download it.

I couldn't believe something this important had gone unnoticed for so long. That paper needed daylight—and I was determined to give it some.

The best $70 I've ever spent. I've joked that it was the down payment on a revolution. Because that one piece of evidence became the snowball that started rolling... and it hasn't stopped since.

Floodgates Open

So I optimized that little website with every search phrase I could think of that matched my desperate, late-night Googling: *eczema treatment not working, eczema worse after steroid cream, red skin after stopping steroid cream, eczema burning and spreading, allergic to hydrocortisone cream, skin flares after steroid use, addicted to steroid cream*—and so on.

And it worked. A torrent began.

Within the first month, letters began pouring in—stories from parents, from young adults, from the elderly, from desperate spouses. They all described the same mystery illness—eerily similar to one another. These were not isolated cases.

Within the first six months, emails came from Canada, Malaysia, Singapore, Japan, England, Scotland, New Zealand, Australia, Ireland, Jordan, India, South Africa, and France. These weren't just letters—they were lifelines. Proof that this was not just my nightmare. It was global. A silent epidemic with no name, no roadmap, and no warning label.

But now we had each other. We had Dr. Rapaport. And we had the truth.

Of the hundreds of letters that poured in, this one captured the heart of what the movement was becoming—not because it was more dramatic, but because it reflected the global awakening that was taking shape. A cause that had quietly crossed oceans. A ripple becoming a wave.

Letter from Karen H. — Queensland, Australia

May 5, 2012

Dear Kelly and Dr. Rapaport,

I'm writing to thank you both from the bottom of my heart. In July and August of 2011, I was enduring intolerable pain and discomfort from a burning, red, inflamed rash on my face, neck, and arms. I felt hopeless and completely alone.

Then I discovered AddictedSkin.org. Through the website—and the generous free link to Dr. Rapaport's research articles—I finally understood what was happening to me: I was suffering from Red Skin Syndrome.

Soon after I stopped steroids, my condition rapidly worsened. The rash spread over my entire body, and I was confined to bed for three months. I had finally quit steroids. During that time, I leaned heavily on the support of the Google Group forum "Cure Eczema by Stopping Steroids," the international community you had created. The only way to overcome Red Skin Syndrome was to stop using topical steroid creams and allow my skin to heal itself. Without the support and shared experiences of others in the forum, I don't know how I would have made it through the darkest days.

I especially appreciated the personal encouragement you both have sent me during that time. Even brief messages meant so much when I was barely holding on.

I reread Dr. Rapaport's articles countless times and made photocopies for family, friends, and even medical professionals. For the first time, I had a clear, science-backed explanation—written by a brilliant dermatologist—to show people who were witnessing my suffering. That alone brought me so much peace.

Kelly, I also want to thank you for organizing and promoting the international teleconferences with Dr. Rapaport and forum members. These calls being freely available on the website became lifelines. Listening to others ask questions—and hearing Dr. Rapaport speak about the condition and its recovery path—gave us all clarity, courage, and a deep sense of connection.

Without the Addicted Skin forum, I would never have known that people all over the world were going through the same thing. Now, I have a global community I can lean on, day or night. I'm no longer isolated in this battle—and that's thanks to you.

It's now been eight months since I found the website, and I'm so happy to report that I'm about 80% healed. The journey hasn't been easy—some days are still hard—but thanks to your unwavering commitment, and to the early support from what is now ITSAN, I've found the strength to keep going.

Thank you both for your tireless work, your generosity, and your belief in the truth.

Warmly,
Karen H.

Karen's story was one of the first... but far from the last. Reading her words, I could feel the distance between us—half a world away—and yet, the same fire under our skin, the same stubborn hope, connected us. Her letter was proof of what I already suspected: this was bigger than me, bigger than my country, bigger than anything I could fight alone. The suffering was everywhere, and so were the fighters.

The letters kept coming—each one a cry for help, each one a match struck in the dark.

From 2009 to 2012, I was still in the thick of my own healing, often answering emails through tears and scratching. *AddictedSkin. org* had become the internet face of a growing underground community, and the Google Group, "Cure Eczema by Stopping Steroids," was our heartbeat.

In the middle of all this, I traveled to California to meet Dr. Rapaport—not once, but four times in two years. I was sick, with raw skin, and often barely functional, but I needed to meet the man whose research had saved my life. We developed a close friendship built on a shared mission: to get the truth out.

Together, we began hosting international teleconferences for patients—calls that gave people real-time access to the only dermatologist openly speaking the truth about Red Skin Syndrome. Those calls were groundbreaking. They connected strangers across continents and turned isolation into solidarity.

This wasn't just about sharing stories anymore. It was about organizing them. Giving this movement structure. Language. Legitimacy. We needed more than a website. We needed a home. A banner to unite under. A place where sufferers could find not just information, but identity, support, and advocacy.

Eventually, we knew the time had come to make it official.

The Spouse Effect

Mark and I boarded a plane from Florida to Los Angeles—me wrapped in layers, skin inflamed, heart pounding with both purpose and pain. Wait—I need to pause here and talk about Mark.

According to a 2015 analysis published in the *Journal of Health and Social Behavior*, the risk of divorce increases when a spouse experiences a chronic illness. Spouses and caregivers are often the little-discussed casualties of TSW.

Mark has been my unwavering support through every step of my journey with Topical Steroid Addiction and Topical Steroid Withdrawal. He was right there with me during the darkest times—through my addiction, my painful withdrawal, and every advocacy effort we undertook together. Remember, this is the guy who allowed himself to be covered head to toe in stinky anti-parasite "goo" for one of the least romantic nights of our lives. Mark puts the "S" in supportive. He accompanied me to visit Dr. Rapaport, sat through countless meetings with doctors, and even lobbied on Capitol Hill and at AAD conferences for ITSAN's mission. Beyond that, he's been my rock, never faltering in his commitment to me.

We've been married for over 20 years, and much of that time has been overshadowed by my chronic skin issues. Mark has missed out on many activities we once enjoyed together, often hearing "not today, honey," due to my struggles. **While we're well aware of the suffering that those with TSA and TSW experience, it's just as important to recognize the toll it takes on their families and loved ones.** Many marriages, like those of two of my close ITSAN friends, have ended because of the strain this condition places on relationships. I'm incredibly grateful that Mark stuck by me through it all, and now, as I'm finally healed, I know the depth of his love and sacrifice. He's suffered too, and I am forever thankful for his enduring support.

Mark's impact has gone beyond our marriage. He's had a profound ripple effect on ITSAN, offering both emotional and financial support. His unwavering dedication has been integral to ITSAN's ongoing work, and without his commitment, I would not have been able to give my full attention to the organization. He has generously donated funding throughout the last 15 years, always saying, "happy to help," because he believes in the cause. His contributions, both in terms of time and resources, have been vital to ITSAN's success and long-term impact. You might catch him wearing one of his favorite T-shirts that says, "What's causing your worsening eczema?"

Okay, now that you know who Mark is, let's go back to the story.

Mark and I boarded a plane from Florida to Los Angeles—me wrapped in layers, skin inflamed, heart pounding with both purpose and pain. It was December of 2011, and we were flying across the country to meet with Dr. Marvin Rapaport. The mission was clear: the movement was growing, and it needed structure. A name. A body. A heartbeat.

The Founding of ITSAN

We gathered at the Beverly Hills home of one of Dr. Rapaport's generous friends. The room was elegant—sunlight streamed through massive windows framing pristine gardens. We sat around a large round table, the kind you'd expect at a strategy summit, not the birthplace of a grassroots revolution. Dr. Rapaport was there, calm and resolute. Mark was beside me, always my anchor. Two of Dr. Rapaport's family members—both doctors themselves, dermatologist Vicki Rapaport and Mathew Torrington, MD—rounded out the group.

There was no debate about the urgency. The stories, the letters, the cries for help from around the world had made it undeniable: this wasn't just a cluster of isolated cases. This was a crisis. We needed an organization to hold it all—every story, every sufferer, every ounce of truth.

We tossed around name ideas. Something global. Something clear. Something that would carry weight.

When we landed on the International Topical Steroid Addiction Network, the room went still.

That was it.

We all nodded. And when we said the acronym aloud—ITSAN— it felt right. Strong. Real. A word that could stand on its own. A word that could carry a cause.

By this point, Dr. Rapaport had seen firsthand the fire in my belly and how hard I had been working—running the Google Group, answering emails around the clock, scheduling teleconferences, maintaining AddictedSkin.org, and supporting sufferers through my own withdrawal. **Always generous, he insisted that I serve as ITSAN's first president and co-founder.** I was honored, and determined to give it everything I had.

Within a year, the group had grown to over 1,000 members across 22 countries. Over 30 new blogs and websites emerged directly from this original community—proof of both the need and the courage to speak out.

Among these early pioneers was Joey Brown, now Joey Van Dyke, who launched the first-ever blog dedicated to Topical Steroid Addiction and Withdrawal. She called it *Red Skin Syndrome*, and it became a beacon for others—reaching hundreds of sufferers and guiding them to Dr. Rapaport's research and healing protocol. Besides her blog, Joey spent hours moderating a growing forum of sufferers and was always available and passionate to do whatever was necessary for the cause. Joey Van Dyke went on to become the second President of ITSAN.

Across the world in Australia, another breakthrough voice emerged. Pete Dawson, whose wife was enduring a brutal withdrawal, created a site that chronicled her healing journey in real time. His writing was raw, honest, and deeply practical—and it struck a chord. His blog soon became the second most-visited TSA/W website in the world, leading countless others to answers they couldn't find anywhere else.

Alongside Joey Brown and Pete Dawson's trailblazing blogs, three powerhouse women emerged as what many in the community came to call the "queen bloggers" of TSW. Louise Jones from the UK, Juliana (who used only her first name, but posted some of the first before-and-after pictures of TSW), and Loren McCormac (who documented her son Kline's skin journey) each chronicled their experiences with brutal honesty, scientific curiosity, and emotional courage. Loren went on to be an ITSAN board member, top advocate and donor. These women's blogs became havens for sufferers around the world—places to learn, vent, cry, and, most importantly, to hope.

By 2014, each of these blogs had amassed nearly 300,000 hits, accounting for well over a million visits combined. And that was just three sites. The internet had become our loudspeaker. What started as whispers in forums and private messages was now a global chorus, echoing with truth.

The Scratchy Monster

Between 2012 and 2013, a group of ITSAN volunteers brought to life something extraordinary—a children's book that gave a face to the invisible monster of TSW. *Taming the Scratchy Monster* was the first of its kind. More than just a book, it was a lifeline for families: a gentle, empowering way to help kids understand what was happening to their skin—or to their parents'.

The idea for the Scratchy Monster was born from the imagination of Keira Ventura, a brave young girl who had survived TSW herself, and grew into a cross-continent collaboration. While still healing from the syndrome, Louise Jones of the UK penned the story. Gloria Pineiro illustrated the whimsical-yet-wise creature that so many kids would come to recognize. And Kristina Ventura, driven by her daughter's journey, edited and produced the book to completion in the United States.

Together, they created more than a story—they created a language for healing. And in the spirit of true community, the rights to *Taming the Scratchy Monster* were given to ITSAN, renewable each year, to help the message reach even further.

Another cornerstone of this grassroots movement was Susan Ryza—a foundational volunteer and one of Dr. Rapaport's earliest TSW patients. Living in Southern California, Susan became a local anchor for the growing number of skin friends who made the pilgrimage to see Dr. Rapaport in Beverly Hills. She and her husband, Steve, opened their home with extraordinary generosity, offering comfort, meals, and a sense of belonging to those in the thick of suffering.

In 2013, Susan took her commitment one step further. She organized and hosted ITSAN's first-ever patient gathering in Los Angeles. It was the first time many of us had met in person after years of online connection. Dr. Rapaport spoke directly to the crowd, and as ITSAN President, I had the privilege of handing out the inaugural Volunteer of the Year Awards to Susan Ryza, Joey Brown (Van Dyke), Kristina Ventura, and Louise Jones.

There were about thirty people in that room. Thirty brave souls in various stages of TSW—adults, children, parents, caregivers. It looked like a room full of the walking wounded: red, swollen, inflamed skin; blankets wrapped tightly; ice packs clutched. Some could barely sit still, the itching was so unbearable.

But then came a moment I'll never forget.

Dr. Rapaport stood calmly at the front of the room, his voice steady and compassionate. He told us we would heal. That this nightmare would end. That our bodies were not broken—they were in the process of mending.

I looked around the room as he spoke and saw dozens of people scratching—arms, legs, faces. The relentless, bone-deep itch of TSW is like no other. But for the first time, we weren't alone in it. We were together. We were seen. We were comforted—by Dr. Rapaport's calm assurance, and by seeing other people who looked like ourselves.

In that Los Angeles living room, listening to Dr. Rapaport calmly assure us we would heal, I realized the mission was bigger than any one of us. We weren't just patients anymore. We were a movement. And even in the darkest times, we managed to find light. Our community's bonds—formed through pain and suffering, advocacy and activism—were gaining momentum.

||||||||||||||||||||||||||||||||||||||||||||||||||||||||||||||||||||||||||||||||||||||||||||||||||||||||||||||||||||||||||||||||||||||||

References

1. Rapaport MJ, Rapaport V. *The red skin syndromes: corticosteroid addiction and withdrawal. Expert Rev Dermatol.* 2006;1(4):547–561. (Nitric oxide rebound and vasodilation mechanism).

2. DermNet NZ. *Topical corticosteroid withdrawal.* https:// dermnetnz.org/topics/topical-corticosteroid-withdrawal (Mechanisms: receptor dysregulation, barrier effects, cytokine cascades).

3. Hengge UR, Ruzicka T, Schwartz RA, Cork MJ. *Adverse effects of topical glucocorticosteroids. J Am Acad Dermatol.* 2006;54(1):1–15. (Systemic endocrine and pediatric HPA-axis suppression).

4. Hajar T, Leshem YA, Hanifin JM, Nedorost ST, Lio PA, Paller AS. *A systematic review of topical corticosteroid withdrawal ("steroid addiction"). J Am Acad Dermatol.* 2015;72(3):541–549. (Notes lack of formal recognition and need for research).

5. Sheary B, et al. *Topical Steroid Withdrawal: A Two-Year Prospective Study of Quality of Life in Adults Ceasing Long-Term Use. Dermatitis.* 2021;32(6):406–414. (Recovery commonly takes 2–5 years).

6. Rapaport MJ, Lebwohl M. *Corticosteroid addiction and withdrawal in the atopic: The red burning skin syndrome. Clin Dermatol.* 2003;21(3):201–214. (Factors influencing recovery: potency, duration, route of administration).

7. Fukaya M. *Topical steroid addiction in atopic dermatitis. Drug, Healthcare and Patient Safety.* 2014;6:131–138. (Describes hallmark symptoms: burning, redness, hypersensitivity, flaking, systemic impact).

CHAPTER ELEVEN

BIRTH OF A MOVEMENT

||||||||||||||||||||||||||||||||||||||||||||||||||||||||||||||||||||||||||||||||||||||||||||||||||||||||||||||||||||||||||||||||||||||||||||||||||||||||||||||||||

ONE OF THE MOST PRECIOUS GIFTS that emerges from the Topical Steroid Withdrawal Syndrome community is the deep, unshakable friendships we form—bonds forged through mutual pain, resilience, and the profound experience of being unseen by doctors but fully seen by each other. It's the kind of camaraderie veterans and cancer survivors might recognize—born not of choice, but of shared suffering.

In moments when crying felt inevitable, we sometimes chose to laugh instead. We sent each other photos of the absurd things we did to stay comfortable—odd clothing, strange positions, makeshift remedies.

The Itch From Hell

The worst part for many of us going through TSW was the maddening itch—the kind that hijacks your nervous system and turns your bed into a battlefield. Bone deep.

Okay, how many times have you already heard me talk about the itch? Sorry—it cannot be overstated. So, we laughed about it.

One forum member once wrote, "As I was trying to sleep last night, I swear to you, if Satan had showed up and asked for my soul in exchange for stopping the itch, I would have said yes!"

Another posted a short video singing along to the Pat Benatar song *Love is a Battlefield*, changing the lyrics to: "My bed is a battlefield, whoa, whoa, whoa, my bed is a battlefield!"

We got creative.

I once bought a real pair of boxing gloves—the kind that requires another person to lace you in. My husband cinched them tight one night, and I went to bed feeling oddly hopeful I'd finally outsmart myself.

But no. In the middle of the night, I managed to untie them using my teeth and got both gloves off, scratching like a maniac, my sheets covered in blood in the morning.

And then there was Tracy Lynn. One of the first people I knew who became addicted to topical steroids through simple over-the-counter 1% hydrocortisone, Tracy's withdrawal was brutal—his mental health frayed and his itch was the worst.

But he still found a way to make us laugh. One day, he sent me a photo of himself that hit my screen and cracked me up until my stomach hurt. He had rigged up plastic dog-cone protectors—yes, the kind veterinarians use after your dog's surgery so it won't bite its wound—and strapped them to the ends of his arms like giant satellite dishes. He looked like he was either trying to contact another planet or cosplay as a crab.

That image lives rent-free in my mind—a symbol of our collective creativity, humor, and refusal to let suffering steal every shred of joy. Tracy later became one of the first male patients to serve on ITSAN's Board of Directors, a quiet pioneer whose intelligence, generosity, and epic sense of humor helped shape the movement.

The First TSA Film

Before there were documentaries. Before there were hashtags. Before the world began to truly grasp the magnitude of Topical Steroid Withdrawal... there was a short film.

And behind that film stood a woman still in the throes of healing.

Jessica Houghton, a Los Angeles-based actor, writer, and educator, never set out to become a spokesperson for a global health crisis. She just wanted her life back. For over 15 years, she'd been prescribed topical steroids—from infancy through adulthood. As her skin worsened and her body unraveled, the only solutions doctors offered were more potent drugs, applied more often. By her late teens, Jessica was searching for answers, but nothing worked—no natural remedies, no prescriptions, no therapies.

Until one desperate Google search changed everything.

She typed: *Can you be addicted to topical steroids?*

That's when she found ITSAN. And her real healing began.

Jessica's journey was anything but linear. By the time she discovered the truth, she was pregnant with her first child—and made the terrifying, empowering decision to withdraw from all steroids cold turkey. Her withdrawal was severe. Her skin bled, peeled, and oozed for over a year. She lost most of her hair. There were no comfort drugs, no shortcuts—especially during pregnancy. It was a raw, exposed time in every way. But like so many others, she clung to the truth... and to her community.

In 2013, not long after ITSAN's formation, Jessica transformed her pain into purpose. She wrote, narrated, and produced *The Dangers of Topical Steroids*, a five-minute animated and live-action film that explained, with striking clarity, the condition now known as Red Skin Syndrome. The film wasn't fancy or high-budget. It was heartfelt, informative, and urgently needed. At the time, it was the only video resource on the internet addressing the iatrogenic condition of

TSA/TSW. It has since garnered over 120,000 views and been translated into several languages, helping countless sufferers understand what's happening to their bodies—and giving them hope.

Jessica's baby was just two months old when filming began. Her husband, an editor and animator, juggled stroller duty while friends like makeup artist Maria Tvdry helped cover flaring skin so Jessica could face the camera. There were moments—many—when, as she put it, "my face had to be literally glued back together between takes." For Jessica, it was chaotic, humbling, and deeply human.

But the result was magic.

Her collaborators—David Bacon (cinematography), Fernando Ontiveros (animation, editing), and Maria Tvdry—brought skill and soul to the project. Together, they created a visual legacy that continues to educate and inspire.

The film gave ITSAN visibility in its infancy and gave patients a voice when few dared to speak. And though Jessica has moved forward in life—now fully healed—her message remains etched in digital stone.

When asked what she would say to someone just discovering they might have TSW, Jessica doesn't hesitate:

"Every tunnel ends in light. And you don't have to go through it alone."

Jessica's film had given our community a voice and a face. But we knew that emotion alone wouldn't change the system. To convince the medical establishment, we needed more than stories and sympathy—we needed numbers.

The First TSW Patient Survey

In 2014, ITSAN board member Dr. James Parker—a medical doctor with quiet brilliance and deep empathy for patients—set out to bring science and structure to what had long been dismissed as anecdotal suffering. He developed and launched a benchmark survey for those affected by Topical Steroid Addiction and Withdrawal Syndrome. It was the first of its kind.

This wasn't just a questionnaire. Dr. Parker, a savant with spreadsheets, built one that crunched a multitude of variables. It became a tool of validation. After completing the survey, participants received two scores: the COSTEX score (Corticosteroid Exposure) and the WAR score (Withdrawal and Recovery). These weren't gimmicks. They were designed to function like medical benchmarks. Just as a person knows their cholesterol or blood pressure, sufferers could now point to numbers that quantified their experience. They could track and share their steroid usage over time.

Dr. Parker's vision was bold. With enough data, researchers might one day be able to correlate the extent of corticosteroid use with the length and severity of withdrawal. Imagine knowing ahead of time how long the road to healing might be. Imagine having the numbers to show a doctor—to defend your decision to stop the creams, to prove that what you were going through was real, possibly predictable, and certainly a tool to avoid more steroids.

Over 3,000 TSW patients filled out the survey. The data was eventually turned over to a handful of researchers and distilled into a poster study presented at the 2015 American Academy of Dermatology Meeting in San Francisco. Researcher Dr. Tim Berger, from UCSF, and Pam Friedman presented the work, entitled *Analysis of Patient-Reported Symptoms With Respect to TCS Usage: A Self-Identified Cohort of Patients With RSS/TSA/TSW*.

This type of survey also became the precursor to ITSAN's future patient registry initiative. Dr. Parker's survey was one more step toward legitimacy. It was a way to make the invisible visible—to give doctors a language they could understand. But credibility alone wouldn't keep the lights on.

Funds From Friends

Before there was crowdfunding, before GoFundMe links and social media campaigns, building a movement still cost money. Even in a volunteer-powered organization, change isn't free. As ITSAN took its first steps, we faced the practical realities of running a nonprofit: website hosting and development, legal and IRS filing fees, conference booth fees, insurance, email and communication tools, graphic design, printing brochures, bookkeeping, and travel to expos and meetings where we could spread the word. Every outreach effort came with a price tag. Traveling to Capitol Hill to lobby for warning label reforms and national awareness days became an annual event.

In those earliest days, we didn't have grants. We didn't have sponsors. We had each other—and a handful of generous believers who dug into their own pockets to light the fuse.

We called them our Top Skin Friends.

These were the donors whose significant startup contributions helped us lift ITSAN off the ground and into the world: Dr. Marvin Rapaport and Jane Jackson; Kelly and Mark Palace; Dr. James Parker and Maria Parker; Kristina and Andrew Ventura; Tracy Lynn; Susan and Steve Ryza; Michael Cernovich; Loren McCormac; Leslie Mahley; and Geanna Bell.

They didn't just give money. They gave trust. They gave belief. They gave the first "yes" in a world full of no.

Their gifts paid for the infrastructure that would support thousands. The ripple of their generosity is still moving today.

It was these volunteers who set up the framework—building the scaffolding of what would soon become ITSAN. Fueled by the momentum of a passionate grassroots army, ITSAN's early years lit up like a spark on dry timber.

What started as a handful of skin-scorched sufferers had grown into a digital uprising—two sprawling Facebook support groups, with over 12,000 members combined, became lifelines to the TSA/TSW community around the globe. Posts flew day and night, in every time zone, filled with pictures, protocols, prayers—and most of all, proof. We weren't crazy. We weren't alone.

Stepping Up The Game

ITSAN was awarded Gold Star status by GuideStar in 2013, the top watchdog for nonprofit transparency. To donors, this was a green light. To us, it was oxygen. Within a short time, we'd garnered more than 100 five-star reviews from patients and parents who'd found not just answers, but hope—a digital trail of healing.

That digital trail of healing was proof we were no longer an invisible community—but we were still outsiders. We'd built our own support systems, our own language, our own credibility with patients. Now it was time to step into the rooms where decisions were being made.

Brush with Arrogance: "Dr. Curls" in Denver

In 2014, we were invited to join the Coalition of Skin Diseases (CSD), a national alliance of patient-led skin nonprofits. These meetings gave us a peek behind the curtain—valuable insight into how other small groups were navigating the complexities of legitimacy, funding, and survival. But the real gift of this affiliation was access. Suddenly, ITSAN had a seat at the American Academy of Dermatology's annual convention—the big leagues of dermatology. The same arena that had long ignored, dismissed, or denied our existence.

That year, Mark and I flew to Denver for the big AAD convention to man the Coalition of Skin Diseases' booth and wave the ITSAN banner in a sea of white coats. But the big part of the trip was that **as President of ITSAN, I was granted five minutes to speak to AAD members about Topical Steroid Addiction and Topical Steroid Withdrawal**. The morning of the presentation arrived, and with it, a knot of anticipation in my stomach. We walked into a large room filled with about fifty doctors, their eyes already fixed on the front. A giant projection screen stood ready, awaiting my words. This was it—the moment to share everything. The facilitator, with her clipboard in hand, began the countdown. "You have five minutes," she said, her voice sharp, the timer clicking to life.

The nerves hit me like a wave, crashing in my chest. This was the big leagues. In swimming, we always say that if you're not nervous before a race, you're not truly ready. It's that surge of adrenaline—the thing that sharpens your focus and drives you to perform. Sure, I get nervous before swim races, but this... this was something else entirely. This wasn't just about a win or loss; it was about people's health, mothers watching their babies suffer in ways they couldn't fix.

My body moved almost instinctively, as if preparing for a race. I found myself doing my pre-race arm loosening, the same little jiggle of my triceps you'd see in Michael Phelps before a dive, that famous flap on the blocks. Every swimmer has their thing. I chuckled softly to myself, thinking how absurdly familiar it felt in the face of such an unfamiliar challenge.

I told myself that if I could just stand up there, deliver my presentation, show them the truth, somehow, this nightmare would be over. The horror would end. I was naive, though, convinced they would listen. But there was no turning back now. With a deep breath, I pushed forward. And told the truth—our truth. When I finished, the room was quiet.

Too quiet.

Then, after my presentation, up waltzed a pediatric dermatologist—head full of bouncy curls, standing well below my eye level, with the confident energy of someone used to thinking they are the smartest person in the room.

With a bright smile and zero hesitation, she said, "With babies, I like to hit them hard with steroid creams at the first sign of a rash."

I stood there stunned. What do you even say to someone who just proudly announced their strategy of pharmaceutical blitzkrieg on infants?

After years of seeing disfigured babies and devastated parents in our forums—victims of that very approach—I'll admit, my blood boiled. I didn't say what I was thinking. I didn't react. These are the battles warriors learn to fight with a smile. Because the truth is, some reckonings don't come with outrage. They come with evidence. And that day is coming.

The fact that she said this moments after hearing my presentation—after hearing the stories, seeing the images, and learning what these drugs can do—was both stunning and clarifying. We weren't just pushing against indifference.

Dr. Curls Cashes In

We were up against arrogance wrapped in clinical credentials. She's the Chair of the Dermatology Department at a major university. Dr. Curls is a made up name, if you haven't already figured that out. I know her real name. I'm not naming her here—frankly, because I'm afraid she might sue me—because she's got more than enough money to sick an attorney on me. She's a bully, plain and simple. She makes a big salary—not just from her university position, but also from drug companies paying top dollar to dermatologists willing to test new drugs on unsuspecting patients. I'm calling her out here because she has likely done more damage to the TSA movement and vocally stood against it, than anyone else.

And if her clinical swagger weren't intimidating enough, like I've just said, her money is too. According to the U.S. government's

Open Payments database, this one dermatologist (whose name I know) has taken over $1.14 million from pharmaceutical companies. That includes nearly $84,000 in general payments, over $57,000 for research fees, and a staggering $1 million in associated research funding—all tied to companies with a financial stake in keeping patients on medication regimens. These aren't obscure backroom checks either. We're talking about Regeneron, AbbVie, Eli Lilly, Dermavant, LEO Pharma, Janssen, and others—the same companies pushing the newest crop of eczema and psoriasis drugs. Source: Centers for Medicare & Medicaid Services. *Open Payments Database* website with the dot gov ending.

When a doctor makes that kind of money from the same industry whose products she's aggressively promoting—especially for little developing pediatric bodies—you have to ask: is this still medicine? Does she even care about these new medicines' long term effects? Or is it just greed in a white coat?

As ITSAN grew, we realized our fight had to be declared away from arrogant doctors, medical dogma, and an industry determined to control the message with its own agenda. We needed to run free in the online streets, race along the hashtag highways, and let the truth of TSW ring out around the digital world.

So strap in—whether you call it warp drive, lightspeed, or folding space, we're about to punch it to the present day. What began as a scrappy little movement is suddenly staring down the big 'B' word of powerful conversations.

CHAPTER TWELVE

SOCIAL MEDIA REVOLUTION

‖‖

TODAY, ON SOCIAL MEDIA, THE HASHTAG TSW on TikTok has soared to 2.2 billion views—that's billion with a "B"![8]

"B" could also stand for Backlash. A backlash against decades of silencing, dismissing, and gaslighting. A backlash against a medical establishment that told sufferers they were rare, hysterical, or simply wrong. TikTok didn't invent TSW, but it made sure it could never be silenced again.[1, 5]

That figure alone is proof of a global health story still absent from official recognition. Fifteen years ago, TSW was a whisper in private messages and forums. Today, the movement has claimed space on TikTok, Instagram, Facebook, Reddit, YouTube, and across the blogging world—not as a vanity trend, but as an act of survival. Patients who once endured in silence have turned their suffering into searchable proof.[1, 2, 7]

This is the social media revolution—not a marketing strategy, but a patient uprising. It's the shift from one-on-one whispers to a global shout, from anonymous symptoms to an identifiable, documented condition.

It's become so powerful that the international leadership of dermatology convened a special meeting just to "combat it." That's the next exposé bonus chapter. But first—what exactly are they trying to combat?

Millions of people are on their phones, in their feeds, telling the truth. Still, one question frames the entire digital awakening: How can videos showing the symptoms of TSW rack up over two billion views online, while the leading U.S. dermatology association, the AAD, offers no prominent public recognition of the condition?[5]

TikTok: The Billions of Views Backlash

When the hashtag #TSW crossed two billion views on TikTok this year, it didn't just break a number—it broke the dam. Millions of people who had never heard of Topical Steroid Withdrawal suddenly saw it in their "For You" feeds: red, cracked skin; oozing limbs; people icing their faces mid-conversation; children in bandages.[8]

TikTok's short-form format turned TSW into a visible, undeniable reality. Survivors posted symptom logs, day-count videos, and recovery milestones that doubled as educational tools. The platform's algorithm pushed these clips far beyond the TSW community, putting them in front of viewers who might never have sought them out. This wasn't passive awareness—it was undeniable.

Rapid Rise: 600 Million to 2.2 Billion Views

In just two years, the TikTok hashtag #TSW soared from 600 million views in 2023, to 1.5 billion in 2024, and as of this writing in 2025, it stands at 2.2 billion.[8] The rise to over two billion in such a short time is more than viral math—it's a cultural signal. And the conversation isn't dying down; the numbers are accelerating.

That growth came from more than just repeat posting. It came from people deciding to join the chorus—newly suffering patients picking up their phones, filming the pain and the progress. It came from comments sections that turned into mini-support groups, from duets and stitches that layered stories on top of one another.

TikTok stats on #TSW (2025): 2.2 billion views, 132,900 videos, averaging 16,800 views each.[8]

If strangers can spot the pattern from a 15-second clip, why can't more clinicians recognize it face-to-face? One woman making a difference is Jenna Romano.

Turning the Camera on TSW

On TikTok, @jennaromano's videos are raw, unfiltered dispatches from the front lines of Topical Steroid Withdrawal.[9] With over 40,000 followers and millions of views, she documents everything—swollen eyes, nights without sleep, the way a Dead Sea salt bath can feel like salvation one day and fire the next. Her captions are frank, her tone conversational, but the effect is surgical: she makes you see what this condition does to a life.

Jenna's TSW journey began in early 2024 after years of eczema treatment spiraled into dependence on topical steroids. When she stopped, the "miracle cream" left her with burning skin, nerve pain, relentless itch, and an unrecognizable reflection in the mirror. Doctors offered only one solution: go back on the drugs. She refused.[6,7]

With no recognition from insurance—and no financial cushion to weather months or years without steady work—Jenna turned to GoFundMe.[10] Her campaign, *Support Jenna's Fight Against TSW,* lays out her economic reality. In it, she calls TSW "the most physically and emotionally devastating thing I've ever endured," a line that, once read, is impossible to forget.

Jenna's online presence is more than personal journaling—it's living evidence. Each video is a timestamped record of injury, recovery, and the refusal to be silenced. In a world where this condition is still dismissed as "rare" or "internet hype," Jenna has turned her phone into both a lifeline and a witness stand.[1, 2, 5]

Instagram: Surge in Reach and Resonance

Instagram gave TSW a different kind of visibility—slower, more curated, but deeply personal. Between 2016 and 2020, #topicalsteroid-withdrawal mentions rose by 288%, and the hashtag's reach—the number of people actually seeing those posts—jumped 592%.[8]

On Instagram, patients could lay their stories out visually: grids showing before-and-after photos, captions unpacking years of misdiagnosis, reels that walked followers through daily care routines. The visual permanence of the platform meant those stories didn't disappear after 24 hours—they stayed, building an ever-expanding archive of evidence.

The hashtags that traveled alongside #topicalsteroidwithdrawal—#thisisnoteczema, #redskinsyndrome, #topicalsteroidaddiction—created a network of connected conversations. Someone searching for one term could stumble into the TSW community almost by accident and find themselves reading post after post that felt like their own diary.[2]

A testament to the epidemic unfolding in children, the Instagram account @ToddlerTSW has drawn 16.7K followers. There, Savannah Jean's mother shares graphic glimpses of her toddler's struggle with topical steroid withdrawal—images of a little one scratching herself raw, her tiny body fighting what was once prescribed as medicine. The account, described as a "mother-daughter duo navigating TSW, advocating, educating, and supporting fellow families," stands as living proof of both the suffering and the growing movement to expose it.[9]

Beyond individual families like @ToddlerTSW, entire networks of advocates are using Instagram to expose the reality of topical steroid withdrawal. Together, these voices represent follower counts ranging from 20,000 to 75,000 each—and collectively, they are approaching half a million people. This digital presence is not just social media; it is a grassroots movement turning private suffering into undeniable public proof. Here is a sampling of some TSW accounts on Instagram:

- @Ctrl.skin — 72K (Instagram) / 346K (TikTok)
- @journey_of_amy (UK) — 52K
- @tsw_renca_czech (Czech Republic) — 15.3K
- @cienarae (US) — 18.4K
- @rocyie (US) — 65.2K
- @_lydslife (UK) — 25.4K
- @eczemawithharrii (UK) — 17.2K
- @remi.tswjourney (UK) — 44.8K (107K TikTok) and Remi has over 21 million views on her YouTube videos.[10]

Cross-Platform Surge: The 274% Boom

Across all major social platforms, mentions of TSW rose 274% between 2016 and 2020.[8] That's not the profile of a niche condition. That's the profile of a public reckoning.

Every repost, retweet, and share pulled the conversation further from the margins. It signaled to patients that they were not isolated cases and to the medical world that this "rare" condition had a growing, vocal, and data-driven community behind it.[2]

And yet, prescriptions for topical steroids—and more potent formulations—continued to rise. Awareness was skyrocketing online, but the system it was calling out wasn't listening.[5]

Reddit: Community Cradle and Crowdsourced Record

While TikTok and Instagram offer mass reach, Reddit offers depth. In forums like TS_Withdrawal, patients trade detailed accounts of symptoms, treatment experiments, and timelines. They post photos not for likes, but for pattern-spotting and shared analysis: *"Has anyone else had this type of swelling at month eight?"* *"Did your ooze stop before or after the redness faded?"*

These conversations form a kind of crowdsourced record—unofficial, but often more detailed than what appears in medical charts. Researchers have even examined Reddit threads in broader dermatology studies, though no conclusive clinical findings about TSW have been drawn from them.[11] Still, the sheer volume of consistent, independent reports raises a quiet but pressing question: How many identical patient accounts does it take before the medical system starts to investigate?[5]

Blogs & Posts: The Written Record of Healing

In 2024, a scoping review cataloged 223 patient-authored TSW narratives—71 blogs and 152 posts across platforms.[12] These stories aren't academic articles; they're raw, often poetic accounts of nights spent awake, skin flaking into the sheets, and the slow, stubborn climb toward healing.

Blogs allow for long-form storytelling—the context, the history, the why. A post might be written mid-flare, or as a reflection years later, but each becomes a permanent entry in the public record of TSW. And when you read enough of them side by side, the patterns emerge—proof by repetition, proof by lived experience.[1, 2]

Facebook: The Quiet Engine of Trust and Support

In a world chasing short-form virality, Facebook remains the backbone of TSW community building.

Private support groups, like those hosted by ITSAN, allow members to speak candidly about symptoms, treatments, and setbacks without fear of public scrutiny. Moderators keep discussions respectful, while members share resources, doctor recommendations, and the kind of encouragement that only comes from someone who has been there.

Public pages—again, ITSAN's page is the leader—extend that conversation outward. They serve as bulletin boards for advocacy updates, legislative wins, and new research, bridging the gap between private suffering and public action.

From Facebook to Academia, these groups don't just comfort—they contribute to knowledge. A 2024 Swedish study on TSW recruited participants directly via a Facebook TSW group and collected detailed patient-reported data.[13] Of 98 respondents, 82 completed the survey, with 95% female, 74% aged 18–39, and 84% self-diagnosed—demonstrating how vital Facebook support communities are in closing research gaps.

The most striking part? This kind of large-scale patient data collection didn't come from public health agencies or major research hospitals—it came from volunteer-run Facebook groups.[5]

YouTube: Where Personal Testimonies Meet Documentary Power

If TikTok is the megaphone and Instagram the scrapbook, YouTube is the archive. It's where TSW stories live in long form—part diary, part documentary, part public record. Search "Topical Steroid Withdrawal" and you'll find everything from shaky-hand confessionals filmed at 3 a.m. to hour-long interviews, skin-care experiments, symptom logs, and expert Q&As.

The reach is substantial. The 10 most-viewed TSW videos on YouTube average nearly 190,000 views each, adding up to millions of plays across the platform.[14] For many newly diagnosed—or self-diagnosed—patients, these videos are the first deep dive into a condition their doctors haven't explained, let alone acknowledged.

But YouTube's value is double-edged. A 2023 analysis of top TSW videos found that while personal narratives dominated, most scored low for reliability and medical accuracy.[15] Only one of the most-watched videos came from a dermatologist, and definitions and timelines for withdrawal varied widely. About half of the popular uploads didn't even use the terms "eczema" or "atopic dermatitis" in the title, underscoring the fractured language around this condition.

That gap creates a vacuum: patients get something to watch; clinicians get little they can cite. And that points to the investigative question: if millions are learning about TSW on YouTube, where are the clear, consensus explanations from major medical bodies—the kind of standardized, public-facing content that could reduce confusion and speed up recognition?[5]

Still, for all its flaws, YouTube remains one of the most influential gateways into the TSW community. Unlike short-form platforms, it allows creators to build trust and depth over time—viewers can follow an entire healing arc, not just a snapshot. It's also where the visual evidence is hardest to dismiss: the gradual change in skin texture, the shrinkage of redness, the regrowth of hair, the return of a smile.[4]

And in that ocean of shaky phone videos, a few works rise above—films with structure, context, and investigative purpose. They don't just show TSW; they argue it. That's where one patient-turned-filmmaker stepped in and changed the game.

Briana Banos – From Survivor to Filmmaker

Her name is Briana Banos—Bri to the community—and she is one of the most visible individuals to put TSW on the digital map. A performer, filmmaker, and truth-teller, Bri transformed her own medical nightmare into two documentaries that would ripple across the globe: *Preventable* and *Still Preventable*.[16]

In 2014, Bri's life looked like it was set to soar. She had just stepped off a cruise ship contract, where she danced and performed for thousands while traveling the world. She'd passed her ACSM personal trainer certification, was in the best shape of her life, and had just married the love of her life in a joyful September wedding. She was happy. She was looking forward to the future.

Then, it all collapsed—"all because of something that was so preventable."[3]

Briana's Descent

Bri had dealt with eczema since childhood, but it had never stopped her from dancing, swimming, or living fully. After the cruise ship job, however, her skin flared harder. A dermatologist, sympathetic at first glance, handed her a prescription for topical steroids. "They worked great—like a true miracle," Bri remembers. But, like so many of us, she quickly learned that the miracle had a timer. The creams stopped working. Her skin flared worse.

As part of the descent, like many who are misdiagnosed, she was given immunosuppressant creams, antibiotics, and antifungals. But stronger steroids were always the doctors' final answer.

After her wedding, Bri decided to stop all of it. That's when the bottom fell out. Her list of symptoms reads like a medical indictment:

- Swollen eyes
- Redness spreading over her body
- Dangerous temperature swings and chills
- Rapid heartbeat and low blood pressure
- Lymph nodes like marbles
- Hair falling out
- "Insatiable itch" that made movement exhausting
- Thick ooze that stuck to her clothes and sheets

This was classic Topical Steroid Withdrawal—iatrogenic, preventable, and devastating.[1, 3]

The Turning Point

"That was the day I decided to do something—to not let this pain go in vain."

Bri turned to YouTube, posting unflinching footage of her skin and her reality. She spoke on national television. She stormed Washington, D.C., lobbying lawmakers on Capitol Hill to recognize the reality and dangers of TSW. She has attended many conferences and expos around the world, even sharing her lived experience through workshops, talks, and workgroups composed of eczema patients, medical professionals, and organization leaders. She has most likely interviewed more patients and medical professionals on this subject than anyone else, asking tough questions about patient care. Again and again, she has seen how dismissive medical professionals can be—but she presses on.[5]

In 2017, Bri crowdfunded a 56-day solo trip around the world to interview fellow sufferers, families, and doctors for what would become the first full-length documentary on the condition.[16]

Preventable (2019) – The First Full-Length TSW Documentary

Released in 2019, *Preventable: Protecting Our Largest Organ* wove together Bri's personal journey with global narratives from TSW sufferers. Filmed over nearly two years, it featured interviews with patients, families, and medical experts—and she traveled to multiple countries to show the universality of the condition.[16]

The film's title spoke its truth: this suffering should never have happened. *Preventable* depicted the physical toll—oozing, swelling, months and years of skin failure—while also exposing the emotional wreckage: lost careers, fractured relationships, and lives on hold. In its first four days, the documentary drew over 12,000 views, quickly becoming required viewing in TSW support circles. The National Eczema Association called it "deeply moving," and ITSAN president Kelly Barta praised it for "depicting the shocking severity of this condition, how widely it affects people, and the urgency of addressing it."[16]

Still Preventable – The Sequel and the Warning

In 2024, Bri returned with *Still Preventable*, a follow-up that showed the crisis hadn't eased. If the first film asked "How can this be happening?", the second demanded, "Why is it still happening?"[3] It explored the persistence of medical denial, the crushing weight on parents of affected children, and the grassroots activism still fighting for recognition.[16]

Distributed freely on her YouTube channel, *Still Preventable* aimed to reach those who needed it most: newly suffering patients looking for answers, and clinicians willing to listen. Viewers described it as "life-saving" and "the only thing that made me feel seen" during the darkest phases of withdrawal.

A Life Rewritten

Bri's story didn't end with the release of her films. TSW didn't just take her health—it reshaped her path entirely. The performer who once danced on cruise ships found herself behind the camera, spot-lighting truths instead of routines.

Feeling "stagnant and misaligned with her life's purpose," she took a bold leap: relocating to Edinburgh, Scotland, to pursue a Master's in Film Directing for Documentary work at the University of Edinburgh. This move was more than a change of location—it was a commitment to mastering her craft. In Edinburgh, she immersed herself in a creative community, navigating the vulner-ability of chronic illness while honing the skills to tell powerful, evidence-driven stories.

Her dissertation project, *Tethered*, is a short documentary ex-ploring the lived experience and fluctuations of chronic health—

an artistic echo of her own journey through TSW. Now embedded in both academia and advocacy, Bri works at the intersection of film and medicine, building a legacy that bridges healing and storytelling.

Preventable remains a milestone in the movement—the first visual document to piece together patient stories into a global narrative. *Still Preventable* carried that work forward, proving the crisis is far from over. Together, they have arguably brought more public attention to TSW than any other single creative work.[16]

Bri's pivot from performer to filmmaker is the clearest possible proof of TSW's impact—not just on skin, but on lives. She turned the loss of one dream into the pursuit of another, and in doing so, she has preserved the truth in moving images for the next generation of patients, advocates, and—if they choose to watch—dermatologists.[1]

As she says in *Preventable*: "If you're in the same position as me... you cannot give up. You cannot. You cannot give up."

Her story doesn't just honor the resilience of those who endure TSW. It makes the condition undeniable.[1]

What Does Briana's Future Hold?

Briana Banos is living proof that a single determined voice can start a wave. What began as one woman, one camera, and a refusal to stay silent has grown into two globally watched documentaries, advocacy on Capitol Hill, appearances at eczema expos and conferences across continents, and even a legislative win in her home state.[16]

Bri's passion for advocacy is contagious—so much so that her mother, Tamy Bellis, joined the fight. They secured a landmark recognition in Florida in 2023: the designation of February 3rd as Topical Steroid Awareness Day—the day ITSAN was founded in 2012. For Bri and her mother, that date now serves as both a rallying point and a reminder that persistence in advocacy can move the needle.[16] And Tamy has lobbied on Capitol Hill for TSW as well.[5]

Preventable and *Still Preventable* documentaries are the kind of work that, one day, may see the same industry accolades given to Hollywood's great documentarians. And in fact, the movement has already drawn the attention of such a figure. From the grassroots urgency of Bri's films to the polished lens of an Oscar-nominated director, the fight against TSW is now being told on screens of every size.

When Hollywood Turns Its Lens on TSW

Enter James Keach—a filmmaker with a career built on telling stories the world needs to hear, and a man whose latest work, *Skin on Fire*, brings the same condition Bri has been championing but with Hollywood experience.[17]

Keach is not a man who wanders into a story without reason. For decades, he's made a career of following the threads of the human condition, pulling them taut until the truth is impossible to ignore. He's played roles in front of the camera, produced the Golden Globe–winning *Walk the Line*, and directed music documentaries for legends like Linda Ronstadt and David Crosby. His Oscar-nominated, Grammy-winning *Glen Campbell... I'll Be Me* didn't just tell the story of a country music icon's battle with Alzheimer's—it invited the world into the fight.

When Keach heard about Topical Steroid Withdrawal Syndrome, he recognized the pattern: a devastating condition hiding in plain sight, dismissed by those in power, endured by those without a voice.[1, 5] He also recognized something else—he'd been prescribed topical steroids himself for poison oak. That personal brush with the drug made the suffering he saw in others feel uncomfortably close. It was enough to light a fuse.

The Making of *Skin on Fire*

In 2022, Keach released *Skin on Fire*, a 29-minute documentary short that plunges the viewer into the lives of people living through TSW.

The stories are raw—patients from all walks of life describing skin so red and burning it feels lit from within, bodies shutting down, careers lost, relationships strained. Their voices aren't staged. They're the unvarnished truth, framed with Keach's cinematic precision.[17]

Alongside these survivors are the medical voices—TSW experts like Dr. Marvin Rapaport and Dr. Peter Lio—explaining exactly what this condition is, how it develops, and why so many patients are trapped in it.[6, 17]

The film walks a careful line: it validates lived experience while grounding it in medical context, the very balance so often missing in the broader conversation. And as of the writing of this book, *Skin on Fire* has over 140,000 views, showing its undeniable reach and impact.

Why It Matters

Skin on Fire is more than a documentary—it's a bridge. In a world of quick TikTok clips and scattered blog posts, Keach's film offers structure, arc, and context. It doesn't just show a rash—it tells a story of cause and effect, of preventable harm compounded by systemic denial.[3]

The film's accessibility matters, too. Keach and his team at PCH Films put it on YouTube, ensuring anyone—patient, parent, or physician—could watch it without a paywall.[17] It quickly circulated in support groups, where viewers praised the director for bringing a neglected condition into the public eye. James Keach's *Skin on Fire* was awarded *Impact Director/Producer of the Year – Body of Work* at the Ethos Film Festival in 2022—a significant nod to its contributions in health storytelling.[17]

Keach's name carries weight in Hollywood and beyond; when a filmmaker of his stature lends his lens to a condition like TSW, it signals that this isn't fringe. This is real. This is urgent.[1]

The Impact

From a purely practical standpoint, the numbers are modest: a short film, under half an hour, quietly uploaded in early 2022. But within patient circles, its impact is outsized. It gives survivors a resource to send to doubting doctors, skeptical relatives, and journalists unfamiliar with TSW. It turns anecdote into narrative and narrative into evidence.[1, 3]

For Keach, *Skin on Fire* is in line with his larger body of work—telling the stories of those who've been silenced, misunderstood, or overlooked.[17] For the TSW movement, it's a turning point. The film is proof that the conversation has climbed out of the support group and into the cultural frame, carried by the kind of cinematic storytelling that can reach people who would never search for "Topical Steroid Withdrawal" on their own.

And that's the quiet genius of James Keach's work. He doesn't just make films. He makes introductions—between a story and the people who most need to hear it. With *Skin on Fire,* he's introduced the world to TSW, and now that we've met, there's no excuse to look away.[1]

Keach's work made TSW impossible to ignore. But the harder truth is this: after the applause dies down, patients are still left to fund their own survival. No safety net. No insurance coverage—because their condition isn't even officially recognized. Just the digital marketplace of desperation—GoFundMe.[5]

The GoFundMe Epidemic

GoFundMe bills itself as "the most trusted online fundraising platform," a digital lifeline where anyone can launch a campaign to pay for what they cannot afford—medical bills, emergency expenses, survival needs. In theory, it's a place for unexpected crises. In practice, for people with Topical Steroid Withdrawal, it has become a public waiting room for the abandoned.[18]

Search "Topical Steroid Withdrawal" on GoFundMe and you'll find something extraordinary—and damning. More active fundraisers appear for TSW patients than the number of patients enrolled in some of the clinical studies used to bring topical steroids to market.[6, 7] That's right: more desperate pleas for help from people injured by the drug than there were participants in the trials that claimed it was safe.

Each campaign is its own case study in suffering and neglect:

- Parents of toddlers who can't sleep for more than an hour without scratching themselves raw.
- Young adults too inflamed to work, watching savings vanish with each rent payment.
- Seasoned professionals forced to move back in with family because the burning and oozing won't let them leave the house.
- Global nomads crowdfunding flights to far-off clinics for treatments like Cold Atmospheric Plasma therapy, because mainstream medicine offers only one "solution": go back on the very drug that caused the problem.

Every GoFundMe page is also a medical record, but one written in the patient's own hand—symptom lists, before-and-after photos, emotional breakdowns at 3 a.m. They're public, timestamped, and searchable. If regulators wanted post-market safety surveillance, they could start here. But they don't.[5]

Harley's Story: The Childhood TSW Stole

One of these GoFundMe campaigns belongs to Harley, a 2½-year-old whose skin has been a battlefield for more than half his life. What began as ordinary eczema spiraled into something far more relentless after months of prescribed steroid creams. When his parents stopped the drugs, his tiny body erupted: constant itching, cracked skin, sleepless nights, clothes sticking to ooze.[1]

Gone were the simple joys—running barefoot in the yard, playing with the family dog, digging in the sand at the beach. For Harley, even a gentle breeze could feel like fire. His mother, Brittany, tried everything within reach: dermatologists, allergists, naturopaths, gut-healing diets, specialized eczema-friendly clothing. But nothing came without cost—financial, physical, or emotional.

Brittany's GoFundMe isn't just about bills; it's about time. Time she can spend caring for Harley without worrying whether they can afford the next appointment, the next batch of medicated bath salts, the next round of special laundry detergent that won't sting his skin. It's about buying back moments of comfort in a young life already defined by pain.[18]

Devastating Finances

Harley is not an outlier—he's the rule.

- **Rebecca, 28** – Once a full-time event planner, now she spends most days in a cold bath to numb the burning. Her campaign is a line-by-line budget for survival: rent, groceries, and enough money to keep her lights on so she can run the fan that makes her skin bearable.
- **Kekoa, 33** – A former Army combat medic, now bedridden. His fundraiser isn't just for his own recovery—it's to get back into ultramarathon shape so he can run races wearing "TSW" across his chest, raising money for the cause he says has taken so much from his own life. He can't work and is asking for living basics.
- **Paola, 41, for Parul** – Paola launched her campaign for her friend Parul, a mother of two who battled TSW for five years before finding CAP therapy in Thailand. The photos on her page are unflinching: Parul wrapped head-to-toe in gauze, her children holding her hand while she sits on the floor, too weak to stand.[18]

Social media gave patients a voice that could no longer be contained. Blogs, films, Facebook groups, and TikTok accounts turned isolated cries into a chorus too loud to ignore. For the first time, the truth about topical steroid withdrawal wasn't hiding in journals or whispered in waiting rooms—it was viral.

And the louder patients became, the more dermatology leadership didn't just notice—they formally strategized ways to discredit, dismiss, and deny. The late-breaking exposé that follows may be the most explosive section of this book. It's time to pull back the curtain.

References

1. Posit #1 — TSW is real.

2. Posit #2 — Prevalence is far higher than admitted.

3. Posit #3 — The harm is real and preventable.

4. Posit #4 — Patterns match globally.

5. Posit #5 — The medical establishment has ignored warning signs for decades.

6. Rapaport MJ, Lebwohl M. *Corticosteroid addiction and withdrawal in the atopic: The red burning skin syndrome. Clin Dermatol.* 2003;21(3):201–214.

7. Fukaya M. *Topical steroid addiction in atopic dermatitis. Drug Healthc Patient Saf.* 2014;6:131–138.

8. TikTok statistics (2023–2025). Hashtag #TSW

9. Romano J. TikTok account @jennaromano.

10. Romano J. *Support Jenna's Fight Against TSW.* GoFundMe campaign (2024).

11. Reddit forums such as TS_Withdrawal.

12. Scoping review (2024). Catalogued 223 patient-authored TSW narratives across 71 blogs and 152 posts. Evidence of recurring patterns and lived experience.

13. Swedish Facebook survey study (2024).

14. YouTube statistics. Top 10 most-viewed TSW videos average ~190,000 views each, totaling millions of plays. (Platform metrics, 2023–2024.)

15. Analysis of YouTube TSW videos (2023).

16. Banos B. *Preventable: Protecting Our Largest Organ* (2019) and *Still Preventable* (2024).

17. Keach J, director. *Skin on Fire* (2022). Awarded *Impact Director/ Producer of the Year – Body of Work* at the Ethos Film Festival (2022). IMDB/PCH Films.

18. GoFundMe platform. Search results for "Topical Steroid Withdrawal" (2023–2025).

DERMATOLOGY LEADERS STRATEGIZE TO FIGHT TSW ONLINE

THEY SAID: *"LET'S SHUT THIS DOWN."* When international dermatology leaders discovered that there were 622 million views and tens of thousands of testimonies appearing online about TSW, they didn't say: let's investigate, but how do we combat this. The online explosion of, now over 2 billion TSW mentions had gotten their attention. **Their own symposium was titled a "cave of misinformation."** Patients were not treated as an opportunity for data, but as a public relations crisis—a swell of voices to be dealt with and silenced.

As patients learn about this symposium, it will land like a double hit. First, the realization that dermatology leaders didn't respond to their suffering with study, but with a strategy to discredit and contain it. Second, if this group of deniers were rattled by 622 million views, today that number is **2.2 billion**—that's a signal you can see from space. And yet the response is to gaslight and retreat back into the "cave," insisting the problem is the voices, not the injury.

Which raises the simplest, most damning question: **Where is the curiosity?** With billions of data points in plain sight—and with some of their colleagues actively treating TSW—why aren't these dermatology leaders, asking what's happening, and designing studies to find out? That is why this chapter is an **exposé**: because what we're seeing isn't science at work, it's suppression by design.

This Was a Training on How to Shut Down the Outcries of TSW Online

And it's all on record. On YouTube, every word, every strategy, every denial is preserved—the voices of dermatology professionals caught planning out their response. Perhaps they never expected anyone to watch closely, or to transcribe their nearly two-hour meeting, word for word. But what follows are their own statements, laid bare. While they did talk about other misinformation in dermatology online, they mentioned the terms topical steroid withdrawal, TSW or red skin syndrome a total of 71 times during the meeting. They lumped a real epidemic in as internet hysteria, calling it an "infodemic."

Source File

International Society of Atopic Dermatitis (ISAD) Online Symposium
Entitled "The Cave of Misinformation"

- 2025 Spring Symposium
- Over 200 dermatology professionals participating
- Held as a video conference
- 1 hour and 54 minutes in length
- Available on YouTube

Source: *Transcript, International Society of Atopic Dermatitis Online Symposium ("Spring Symposium"), Spring 2025.*

Enter the Cave

In April 2025, more than 200 dermatology professionals logged onto a Zoom call hosted by the International Society of Atopic Dermatitis (ISAD). The title of the meeting? *Misinformation in Atopic Dermatitis.*

From the very first words of the facilitator, the tone was clear: *"We are sitting in our cave, the cave of misinformation today."*

This was not a scientific meeting about new research or patient outcomes. This was a strategy session to combat claims of TSW. The enemy was not atopic dermatitis itself—but patients who dared to tell the truth about their own suffering caused by their doctors' treatments.

The Irony of "Misinformation"

Speaker after speaker described patients' lived experiences as though they were viruses to be eradicated.

Direct quotes from the meeting: *"I must say I was not aware how much misinformation is in social media, so I did a little bit of research and I'm really shocked."* **"It is extremely common on social media, but rare in doctor's offices."**

The irony is jaw-dropping. By labeling patient experiences as "misinformation," these physicians invert reality itself. Decades of published warnings, clinical studies, and case series—detailed in the proof section of this book—already establish the patterns of topical steroid addiction and withdrawal across continents. Japanese dermatologists have named it, Indian task forces have campaigned against it, European clinicians have documented it, and American pioneers like Rapaport have published it. The data is there. The global patterns are there. The doctors willing to tell the truth are there. What emerges from this symposium, then, is not an effort to clarify facts but to obscure them. It is dermatology itself generating the misinformation, recasting testimony as hysteria and evidence as rumor.

Sleight of Hand

One speaker even quoted the World Health Organization's definition of misinformation:

"So the World Health Organization has described misinformation as the greatest threat to global health, and in 2016, post-truth was chosen as

the Oxford Dictionary's Word of the Year. Misinformation is an infodemic, otherwise known as an overabundance of information and rapid spread of misleading or fabricated news."

The very description they wield against patients applies most accurately to their own denial. To call social media "the cave of misinformation" is less an analysis than a projection—the professional pot calling the patient kettle black. In that sense, the meeting felt less like science than a descent into a post-truth twilight zone, where denial becomes policy and narrative control replaces inquiry.

Of course it's "rare" in their offices. They don't measure it. They misdiagnose it as eczema. And patients no longer trust them enough to walk through their doors, or listen to their advice online.

Critics of the Medium

Instead of learning about prevalence or discussing patient care, they critiqued the way patients communicated.

"Despite poor quality, their videos had very high reach, high number of views, high number of comments, and high number of shares."

Not a single speaker proposed analyzing this massive dataset for patterns or truth. Instead, they strategized ways to drown it out and shared diagrams showing dermatologists as the only voice that could be trusted and discussed ways to correct all the "poor quality" videos of patients sharing their TSW journey, trying to find help.

Infodemic

To be clear, the symposium did cover other forms of online voices on eczema of what they called "misinformation." One presenter described a literature review that turned up 133 abstracts, only one of which they deemed suitable, and then expanded the search with Google. Their thematic analysis grouped online "misinformation" into buckets: claims of simple eczema cures, dietary triggers, environmental chemicals, dust, vaccines, red skin syndrome, and alternative regimens.

The examples included vegan diets promising to "cure eczema in days," conspiracy theories about formaldehyde or laundry detergents, devices marketed as "dust solutions," and even the suggestion that 5G caused eczema. They also noted homeopathy websites blaming vaccines, exploiting the fact that eczema often appears in infancy around the same time routine vaccinations begin.

In short, they treated everything from diet fads to dust conspiracies to vaccine denial as part of one broad "infodemic."

And into that same hysterical bucket, they placed topical steroid withdrawal—equating the testimony of hundreds of thousands of patients with pseudo-science about 5G, vaccines and detergents.

As one speaker put it: *"Red Skin Syndrome, also referred to as topical steroid addiction or steroid withdrawal, is a controversial and popular topic on TikTok and tabloid newspapers. Proponents of this theory claim that the skin problems are caused by topical steroid addiction."*

By collapsing real injury into conspiracy theory, they didn't just miss the signal—they dismissed it as part of the "infodemic."

The "622 Million"

It came from one doctor's TikTok analysis:

"So these patients on social media share their experiences and we have more than 622 million views on TikTok about this topic. Though it is not formally defined as a separate condition, it is extremely common on social media, but rare in doctor's offices."

This is dynamite because they acknowledge the scale—hundreds of millions of testimonies—and still minimize it as "rare in doctor's offices."

The "Solutions"

Here is where the symposium turned from silence to push-back.

"Healthcare professionals can stop the spread of false information by refuting or rebutting misleading health information."

"We wanna try to reply at least to these very high reach videos... give proper advice and try to reach the same people that look at this hashtag."

1. ***Proposal to use clickbait for attention***

    Dr. Hanof says, *"Maybe we should start with sensational titles like 'How you can cure in two days' instead of saying 'don't be afraid of steroids' because then no one will read it."*

2. ***Anecdote framed as a one-day cure***

    Dr. Hanof says, *"I would post this. I would title it as healing with steroids. A one day success story... And only after one day of using a topical corticosteroid, she had almost complete resolution of her symptoms."*

3. ***Admission it was promotional, though "anecdotal"***

    The facilitator asks, *"Dr. Hanoff, are you promoting the use of TCS for one, only one day?"*

    "Yes... we need to include disclaimers that this is anecdotal evidence. Because this is one patient experience... Not all patients will need one day versus, let's say 10 days and so on," Dr. Hanoff concluded.

This is not medicine. This is marketing. This is truly misinformation. Neither eczema nor TSW can be cured in two days. This is their own post-truth.

Corticophobia as a Scapegoat

When confronted with distrust, they did not ask why patients distrust them. Instead, they diagnosed the distrust itself as pathology:

"70% of patients express fears about TCS... 24% non-compliance because of fears."

"This reveals some significant knowledge gaps."

"Corticosteroid phobia is a worldwide phenomenon... the first scale to assess TCS phobia has good psychometric properties."

In other words: if patients resist steroids, it's not because they've been injured. It's because they're phobic, irrational, and misinformed.

The Real Public Health Crisis

The symposium could have been a turning point. With over 200 dermatology professionals assembled, and millions of patient data points at their fingertips, they could have launched the largest observational study in the history of eczema. They could have asked:

What if the patients are right?

Instead, they asked: *How do we silence them?*

When the largest dataset in dermatology history appeared, they didn't see science. They saw a PR problem.

They are, in fact, late to the party. The 622 million views they fretted over are now 2.2 billion.

The cave of misinformation was their own misinformation—denial rebranded as science. And the next betrayal we look at comes from the very advocacy groups patients thought were on their side.

|||||||||||||||||||||||||||||||||||||||||||||||||||||||||||||||||||||||||||||||||||||||||||||||||||||||||||||||||||||||

PART V

THE RESISTANCE

CHAPTER THIRTEEN

THE SHIELD: PATIENT ADVOCACY GROUPS

EVERY PATIENT WITH TOPICAL STEROID withdrawal is like **a warrior dropped into a video game of TSW Denial** that they never signed up for. The mission is simple: find the truth, find relief. But standing between us and the answers are three levels of defense, each one tougher than the last.

Level One: The Shield. Patient advocacy groups like the National Eczema Association NEA, here in the US, became the first shield of denial—deflecting our voices, muffling our warnings, keeping the medical world from hearing us. They should be amplifying our voices, not blocking them. NEA wasn't the only group to be slow in taking action—most of the eczema groups around the world have behaved the same way

Level Two: The Soldiers. These are the dermatologists. Not neutral exam-room guides, but enforcers of the "standard of care." When patients came in naming their own condition, it felt to them like an intrusion, a usurping of authority. Their response was to gaslight, to dismiss, to shut us down. They became the foot soldiers of denial.

Level Three: The Fortress. Behind it all stands the final boss—the regulators, corporations, and medical associations. In the US, the FDA, meant to protect patients, Big Pharma, built to protect profits, and the AAD, who sets and is the gatekeeper of clinical practice guidelines. Together they form the fortress wall: authority, money, and hierarchy. The doctors don't just act out of ignorance or arrogance; they act because that's how the health ecosystem is set up to work.

This section of the book is about breaking through each level. Chapter 13 takes on the Shield. Chapter 14 faces the Soldiers. And in Chapter 15, we confront the Fortress itself.

Let's start with the Shield—in the world of eczema here in the US, that shield has long been the National Eczema Association (NEA). Back in 2012, when ITSAN and the TSW movement began, instead of protecting patients, it blocked them. Instead of amplifying our voices, it muffled them. For years, the NEA stood as the first line of defense against any acknowledgment of topical steroid addiction (TSA) or withdrawal (TSW).

As this book is being written in 2025, the relationship between ITSAN and the National Eczema Association (NEA) has improved substantially. Like turning the Titanic, progress has been painstaking—but, the ship has finally begun to change course. NEA is now more open to dialogue about topical steroid withdrawal syndrome and the patients it affects. It took years of appeals from patients and caregivers for them to put any helpful information or resources regarding TSA and TSW on their website, and to include education on the condition in their annual patient conference, but they have done it.

Not to Shame but to Shift

However, it's important that we document the full, complicated history between these two organizations—not to shame, but to show how difficult it is to shift systems that are influenced by money, power, and outdated dogma. This is a case study in how truth is resisted, how patients are gaslit, and how a grassroots movement can begin to change the tide.

Since 1988, the National Eczema Association has stood as the largest and most visible patient organization for eczema sufferers in the United States. I even donated money to them and once pitched a fundraising idea called *Itching for a Cure*, a 5K race series I dreamed up as an athlete and race director. I believed they were advocating for people like me.

But in my interactions with them, it became clear that NEA's priorities were heavily influenced by the biases of its medical advisors and pharmaceutical sponsors. In terms of sponsors, a glance at their website confirmed it—the logos of big pharma companies dominated their website like a corporate billboard. This financial entanglement felt like a massive conflict of interest. The very drugs causing harm were funding the organization meant to help us heal.

As the new President of ITSAN in 2012, I reached out to NEA's, then, executive director, with whom I believed I was on friendly terms. I'd spoken to her before as a supporter of NEA. So I picked up the phone and asked if ITSAN could have a small booth at their upcoming Expo—just to provide an alternative perspective. **She didn't just say no. She said she had heard about us and that we were a bunch of "internet conspiracy theorists."** Then she quickly ended the conversation with me. ITSAN's attempts to gain access to the NEA Expo became an annual effort for the first several years. Every year, like a bad sequel, we were denied—not even a polite "thanks but no thanks"—just a firm "not a chance, we don't buy it." So eventually, we gave up and decided there were better ways to reach those who needed our message.

These were some of the most disheartening moments of my advocacy journey. I realized then just how much this Goliath had to lose if ITSAN—the David in this story—turned out to be right.

A Threat to Call Security

That wasn't my first disturbing encounter with NEA or being bullied. During a trip to Los Angeles to see Dr. Rapaport, my husband and I discovered, through the NEA's website, that there was an eczema support meeting at UCLA, focused on treating severe eczema. One of the topics to be discussed at this meeting was the use of wet wraps, which are a way to increase the absorption of topical steroids—by covering the medicated skin in occlusive layers, a practice that is an off-label use and again, according to researchers McKenzie and Stoughton (*Arch Derm*, 1962) occlusion could increase absorption more than 100-fold. This infuriated us. This practice is most commonly done in infants and children, as you will hear in this book from exasperated parents.

But we decided to attend the meeting anyway to bring the valuable knowledge of Topical Steroid Addiction as a possible way to help suffering parents and patients. I remember on our way sitting in LA traffic, having the discussion whether we should turn around or not. We were on East Coast time and the meeting was in the evening, and we were already past our usual bedtime and jetlagged. But knowing we might help just one person find the answer to their pain, we pushed on.

When we arrived, the room was filled with children and desperate parents. Many of the kids had clear signs of Topical Steroid Addiction—the white nose surrounded by inflamed red cheeks, red "sleeves" on the skin of their arms, and pale palms. These are hallmark signs of topical steroid addiction.

When I raised my hand and asked the presenting doctor if worsening eczema might be the result of topical steroid addiction—citing the published work of Dr. Marvin Rapaport—I was shut down. "We're aware of Dr. Rapaport's work," the doctor said. "We don't believe in that." Then I was told if I wanted to discuss that, I'd be asked to leave. When I would not be silenced and tried to explain how I had brought peer-reviewed clinical articles on TSA with me, and I myself was now a healing patient in recovery from TSA, the hostility in the room escalated. A mother shouted, "I arranged this meeting! You need to go!" And next we were threatened with being escorted out when one of the moms asked, "Doctor, would you like me to call security?"

We were being treated like criminals. It was clear: belief in steroid-induced harm was treated like heresy.

The NEA "Pump Fake"

But we weren't alone. Back in San Francisco, Kristina Ventura, a fierce mother whose daughter Kiera was suffering through withdrawal, lived near NEA's headquarters. Yes, the same family that brought the children's book, *The Scratchy Monster*, to life. Kristina visited NEA repeatedly. She brought clinical papers in binders. She printed photos of her daughter's pain. She documented other children suffering in the same way. She was the first patient-advocate who showed up at their doorstep—physically—to challenge their narrative.

Still, NEA resisted. Even Dr. Rapaport himself reached out, many times over the years, but was stonewalled each time.

Eventually, in 2015, under pressure from ITSAN and growing awareness, NEA formed a "Topical Steroid Addiction Task Force" and asked them to produce a review paper on their findings. It sounded promising—like an olive branch.

When I first heard the National Eczema Association was forming a Task Force to investigate Topical Steroid Addiction, something in me lit up. The optimist. The fighter. The woman who had been battling this thing from the frontlines for six years already. I thought— *This could be it.* Maybe NEA would finally embrace the truth. Maybe the silence was ending.

I'll never forget where I was when their findings were announced. Standing in the middle of a Lowe's hardware store in

Florida, dressed in jeans and a long-sleeve shirt in the suffocating heat, trying to shield my raw, broken skin and keep from freezing in 90 degrees—yep, body temperature dysregulation is part of TSW. I wore white cotton gloves with the fingertips cut off—the only way I could use my bleeding, oozing hands. My phone rang. It was Kristina Ventura, who you know by now. Her voice was excited and concerned. "They've posted it," she said. The NEA's findings were live.

I ran out of Lowe's like there was a bomb threat announced. At home, I pulled up NEA's website, hoping for something—anything—that might acknowledge the reality we were living through. As I began to read their findings, my cautious optimism started to slip away. By the time I finished reading the report, I found myself on the floor, forehead pressed to my knees, body trembling as tears fell.

The National Eczema Association had betrayed all the people suffering in silence.

The report was supposed to be a turning point. Instead, it was a gut punch—a reminder that even those who claim to care can look the other way when the truth is inconvenient. Their "review" paper read more like damage control than truth-telling. ITSAN issued a strong response—not out of bitterness, but because too much was at stake.

Here are the five critical failures of their biased paper:

1. **Minimizing the Scope**

   The NEA labeled TSA as "rare"—without sufficient data. They ignored the vast global patient community, the underdiagnosed cases, and the tidal wave of evidence flooding social media, support groups, and clinical practices. Rarity isn't truth when misdiagnosis is the rule. Much like AIDS or Legionnaires disease would have been seen as rare back in the 1980s.

2. **Ignoring Children's Suffering**

   While NEA's paper focused mostly on adult women, our support communities told a different story—filled with suffering children. Ignoring this population was more than a scientific oversight; it was a moral failure. Dr. Fukaya's research papers also told a different story.

3. Cherry-Picked Data

The review omitted cases where steroids were used on common areas like arms, hands, and legs—a deliberate narrowing of the evidence to those that were used on the face. By excluding broader steroid usage, they downplayed the true reach of addiction.

4. Erasing Experts

Notably absent? Dr. Rapaport and Dr. Fukaya—the very pioneers who had treated thousands of patients and published extensively on the condition. Their exclusion wasn't accidental; it was strategic.

5. Conflict of Interest

Perhaps most damning: NEA receives financial support from companies that manufacture topical steroids.

A Missed Opportunity

The National Eczema Association's review wasn't just flawed—it was a missed opportunity. **Why am I bringing up a decade old issue?** Because ten years ago, NEA could've changed the course of thousands of lives. Instead, they buried the truth under politics.. Mothers are still rocking their children through nights of burning skin. Patients are still spiraling in confusion, shame, and pain. And the medical world still shrugs.

They hid the truth because of their agenda, and if that wasn't an obvious shield against going public about TSW, then what happened in 2019 was another clear move to put a hush on TSW awareness.

Not Exactly a Gag Order

In October 2019, TSW survivor Kelly Barta accepted a full-time role with the National Eczema Association (NEA) as Senior Manager of Advocacy. It was a chance to represent the patient voice in a broader way through working with the largest eczema organization in the United States. But upon taking the role, she was told she would need to distance herself from ITSAN and from the issue of topical steroid withdrawal. NEA didn't want their senior advocate to be "known for TSW," even though, as Barta pointed out, roughly 80% of the advocates she worked with were either going through withdrawal or had already survived it. The very condition driving patients to advocacy was the one she was expected not to speak about.

The message was never delivered as a formal gag order, but it was no less clear: she could not openly align with ITSAN, she could not accept invitations to talk about TSW, and she could not let her story—the very reason she was in advocacy—define her work at NEA. When a prominent podcast invited her to share her experience, she ran it past her supervisor, only to be told no. Opportunities to raise awareness were closed off because of her role.

It left her in a murky limbo—no outright ban, but no safety to speak either. "I didn't feel like I could openly talk about it," she explained. And that was the breaking point. The whole reason she had entered advocacy was to fight for and help families navigate through eczema and steroid withdrawal to reclaim their health. If she couldn't do that, there was no reason to stay. She stepped away from NEA, disappointed by an organization that claimed to give patients a voice while quietly censoring which truths could be spoken.

If the NEA was a disappointment, the American Academy of Dermatology was a devastating betrayal. Bigger budget. Louder microphone. An army of white coats united not by curiosity, but by fear—fear of liability, fear of admitting they'd harmed the very patients they swore to protect. If the NEA had simply looked the other way, the AAD actively built the wall that kept TSW out of the conversation. They weren't just slow to recognize the truth—they abandoned the oath of "first, do no harm." And I'd seen that arrogance before.

And this was the next level of the denial game: the soldiers. No longer just a shield of silence, but dermatologists in exam rooms, armed with authority, arrogance and ready to tell patients their condition wasn't real.

CHAPTER FOURTEEN
DEAR DERMATOLOGISTS

IIIIIIIIIIIIIIIIIIIIIIIIIIIIIIIIIIIIIIIIIIIIIIIIIIIIIIIIIIIIIIIIIIIIIIIIIIIIIIIIIIIIIIIIIIIIIIIIIIIIIIIIIIIIIIIIIIII

PICTURE THIS: A PATIENT SITS IN A COLD exam room, feet dangling from the paper-covered table. Their skin is red, cracked, and unbearably itchy. They haven't slept through the night in months. Every movement feels like sandpaper on raw nerves. They are desperate—and hopeful—because any minute now, the expert will walk in. The dermatologist. The person they've been told is the authority, the one who knows how to fix skin.

I know this scene well. I lived it. As I wrote about in *Down the Rabbit Hole*, I sat across from dermatologist after dermatologist— five in a row—while my condition worsened and my questions grew louder. And just like countless patients I've spoken with since, I trusted that the person in the white coat would see my suffering, recognize what was happening, and guide me toward healing.

But that is not what happens.

Root of the Problem

In the preface, I state the root problem of this epidemic: the "experts" are denying that topical steroid addiction (TSA) exists. So when the gatekeepers of medicine and public health—news media, medical journals, the FDA, the eczema associations, insurance companies, the CDC, even parents and patients—ask about TSA, they turn to dermatologists. And the answer is almost always the same: *"This condition does not exist."* Or, if pressed: *"It's a rare reaction." "It's just internet hysteria."* This has gone on for decades.

I have personally been to more than a dozen dermatologists who do not believe in TSA. Being part of the TSW community for the last twenty years, I have spoken with hundreds of patients whose dermatologists told them there was no such thing—and then tried to hand them more steroids. For decades, Dr. Rapaport has been shut out by this same academy, along with the handful of brave TSA-friendly doctors around the world who dared to raise the alarm.

And here is the truth: this epidemic could be slowed with one simple change—revising the prescribing guidelines for skin conditions. If the American Academy of Dermatology—and the equivalent governing associations in other nations—updated their treatment standards, the cycle of harm would end. Because dermatologists always fall back on the same safeguard: *"This is the standard treatment."* When the standard itself is broken, that defense collapses.

Leaders Denying

But it's not just local dermatologists clinging to dogma and hiding behind the "standard of care." It's some of the most visible leaders and voices of authority in dermatology. And let me be clear: these examples of arrogant denial are not secretly recorded or stolen from private documents. They are public-facing statements, delivered on stages, in journals, on podcasts, and across social media—content broadcast for the world to see.

- **Dr. Steven Feldman — Professor of Dermatology, Wake Forest University School of Medicine, North Carolina** — on stage at a large dermatology conference, during a CME session teaching hundreds of physicians never to say the word *steroid.*

- **Dr. Jean-François Stalder — Professor of Dermatology, Nantes University Hospital, France** — lead author of the international *TOPICOP* study, which created a "corticosteroid phobia" score to pathologize patient fears and reframe caution as a diagnosis.

- **Dr. Deshan Sebaratnam — Associate Professor of Dermatology, University of New South Wales, Sydney, Australia** — leveraging his Instagram following to bully and discredit anyone who dares to mention TSA.

- **Dr. Dustin Portela — Dermatologist and social media influencer, Boise, Idaho** — with 156,000 online followers, soothing the public with TSW minimizations.

- **International Society of Atopic Dermatitis (ISAD)** — hosting a 2025 symposium that planned strategies to suppress patient voices about TSW instead of studying them.

Ask any of them, and the denial is loud and clear. These five **voices of authority** are just the tip of the iceberg—a sample of the attitudes on TSA that have dominated dermatology.

To keep things engaging, I've written letters to different "types" of dermatologists in the TSW universe. Each letter is an exhibit, written in the patient's voice—sometimes on behalf of all of us, sometimes as my own. Together, they show the patterns we face: minimization, bullying, dismissal, and, in rare cases, humility.

Exhibit A

Dear Dr. Steven Feldman,

Your words as you stood on stage at a CME symposium in front of hundreds of dermatologists were insulting to patients. You were not in a comedy club, but at a medical conference—and yet this is what you taught your colleagues: never say the word *steroid* to patients. Mislead them with alternative language. Deflect their concerns rather than addressing them.

Here is your own transcript, word for word, as you explained how you dodge the truth when patients ask if a cream is a steroid:

> *"When I'm asked a question I don't want to answer, I just answer a different question. I never use the word 'steroids' in front of patients, ever. I tell them, 'This is an all-natural, organic, anti-inflammatory, designed to complement your natural healing mechanisms to bring the immune system back into balance and harmony.' If they're from Portland or wearing Birkenstocks, I'll add 'gluten-free, made in a nut-free facility.' If they're from middle America and wearing a MAGA hat, I'll throw in 'made in America.' Every word is true—I just don't say it's a steroid."*

Dr. Feldman, you stood before a room of physicians and taught them how to manipulate language, how to dodge the truth, how to deceive the very patients whose trust they hold. Our suffering is not a punchline about Birkenstocks or red hats. Every laugh in that room came at the expense of patients whose lives have been wrecked by the very drugs you were teaching doctors to disguise.

You didn't just fail to give us informed consent—you taught others how to withhold it, too. And as a patient, if I thought something was "all natural and organic," I would use it freely and often, with no concern for harm. Is that your intent?

No wonder dermatologists won't tell patients about the dangers of steroids—they're being taught not even to use the word.

Source: CME lecture, International Investigative Dermatology Conference, Orlando, 2018. *Oculus Virtual Reality Symposium: "New and Emerging Agents for the Management of Moderate-to-Severe Atopic Dermatitis in Adults: A Virtual Reality View."* Transcript from publicly available video on YouTube.

Exhibit B

Dear Dr. Stalder and Colleagues,

You didn't just ignore our concerns about topical steroids. You gave our resistance a diagnosis. You called it "corticosteroid phobia." Let me ask you, how can we be steroid phobic, when most of us have used steroids freely for years? **We aren't steroid phobic, we are steroid informed.**

Instead of helping us, you built a questionnaire—twelve items scored on a four-point scale—and turned our lived experiences of harm into a number you named the TOPICOP score. Then you published it across 17 countries and 21 hospitals, surveying more than 1,500 patients and parents, most of them children or guardians answering on their behalf.

The results were striking: nearly half of respondents worldwide expressed fears or reluctance about topical steroids. The highest scores came from Taiwan, Poland, and Ukraine; the lowest from Japan, Brazil, and Denmark. And the hardest questions for patients to answer? Do steroids pass into the bloodstream? Do they cause infections? Do they cause asthma? Even your own paper admitted there was "conflicting evidence" on these issues.

Yet instead of treating patient fears as a signal that more research was needed, you declared the fears themselves the pathology. Instead of asking why so many parents around the world were afraid, you labeled the parents irrational. Instead of listening to us, you pathologized us. This was not an honest inquiry into harm—it was a study of resistance, dressed up as science.

To call us "phobic" is not to describe us; it is to dismiss us. Phobia is a rhetorical hammer, a way to shut down debate and discredit those asking questions. Once labeled, our words no longer count, our experiences no longer matter, and our pain can be ignored. That may be convenient for you. But it is devastating for us.

If even you admit there is conflicting evidence, how can you call patients phobic for asking those questions? If you cannot agree on the science, why pathologize the skepticism? Imagine if the same collaboration of 17 countries and 21 hospitals had been used to study topical steroid addiction itself, rather than mocking the people raising the alarm. You might have uncovered the truth. You might have saved lives.

When nearly half of your patients worldwide are afraid, that is not phobia. That is a warning. And you ignored it.

Source: Stalder J-F, et al. *Topical corticosteroid phobia in atopic dermatitis: international feasibility study of the TOPICOP score. Clinical and Translational Allergy,* 2017.

Exhibit C

Dear Dr. Deshan Sebaratnam,

Your frequently active Instagram page has over 8,000 followers, most of whom appear to be fellow dermatologists in Australia. As a professor at the University of New South Wales, you undoubtedly influence and train the next generation of physicians. In some recent Instagram posts, you didn't just deny topical steroid withdrawal. You went further. You used your platform to bully and discredit the very people most affected.

DEAR DERMATOLOGISTS

Here are your public posts:

- You mocked an Australian mother whose baby was suffering steroid withdrawal.
- You dismissed the journalist covering her story.
- You reposted the headline—*"Mum says baby's severe skin symptoms are withdrawal from treatment"*—and scrawled across it: *"Based on her own online research."*
- You captioned it: *"Irresponsible clickbait contributing to misinformation of the Australian public."*
- You told your followers: *"If TSW is real, why don't we see it in lupus, lichen sclerosus, or Cutaneous T-Cell Lymphoma?"*

This isn't a medical debate. It's bullying—a tactic to shame parents, to dismiss reporters, to make sure the conversation never gets traction. But intimidation is not evidence.

And your post asking "why don't we see TSW in other conditions?" argument is not logic—it's misdirection. The good Doctor Rapaport answered your misdirection question as follows: lupus, lichen sclerosus, and Cutaneous T-Cell Lymphoma are typically localized, stable, and treated in short courses. Atopic dermatitis is widespread, relapsing, and often treated daily across large body surface areas—especially in children with impaired skin barriers. The difference in exposure explains the difference in outcome. That's not proof against withdrawal—it's precisely why withdrawal emerges in eczema and not elsewhere. *(Clinical references below.)*

You had a choice: to acknowledge the data, or to bully and dismiss those who raised it. You chose to mock a mother and a journalist instead. That may rally colleagues on Instagram, but it leaves patients abandoned.

And I have to wonder: do you think other dermatologists who may privately recognize TSW would ever speak up in your presence? Or does your ridicule keep them silent too?

183

Our suffering is not misinformation. Parents advocating for their children are admirable. Journalists covering a health crisis are not "clickbait." When you call them out, you reveal more about your priorities than theirs.

Source: Dr. Deshan Sebaratnam, public Instagram account, July 19 and July 21, 2025.

Exhibit D

Dear Almost There Dr. Portela,

You did something few of your colleagues have ever had the courage to do: you admitted topical steroid withdrawal is real. For that, patients thank you. In a profession built on denial, you said the words out loud. You even interviewed Dr. Marvin Rapaport—the very man most dermatologists avoid naming, let alone platforming. That took openness, and it mattered.

But then came the hedge.

- "Yes, it's real… but it's rare."
- "There's very little research around this topic."
- "Most of the potential therapies are crowdsourced by patients."
- "The vast majority of people who use steroids as recommended will not have significant problems."

Dr. Portela, this is where your words failed us. Rare means ignorable. Rare means dermatologists can nod sympathetically, then keep prescribing. Rare means patients are still dismissed as anecdotes, left to find each other online while dermatology pats itself on the back for "listening."

And as for research—it is there. Rapaport, Fukaya, Lahiri, Damisetty—dozens of peer-reviewed studies from Japan, India, the UK, and beyond. You called it crowdsourcing only because your field has ignored it. Patients filled the vacuum not because science was absent, but because your journals refused to publish it.

With 156,000 followers, your voice matters. Neutrality is not neutral when you have that kind of reach. Your half-recognition soothes the profession—but still abandons the patients.

You almost get it. You are so close. But until you say it plainly—this condition is not rare, it is iatrogenic, and it is fueled by standard prescribing—your words continue the betrayal.

Our suffering is not "rare." It is not "crowdsourced." It's real.

Source: Dustin Portela, DO, YouTube video "Is TSW Real?", 2022.

Exhibit E

Dear International Society of Atopic Dermatitis (ISAD),

In the spring of 2025, more than 200 dermatology professionals gathered under your banner for a symposium you called "The Cave of Misinformation." The title alone revealed the posture: not curiosity, not humility, not science—but contempt. You treated patient testimony as a virus to contain, a public relations crisis to manage.

You did not say: "Let's investigate." You said: "Let's shut this down." Instead of asking why hundreds of millions of patients are speaking out, you strategized how to bury their voices. Instead of launching the largest observational study in eczema history, you proposed clickbait "two-day cure" stories to compete with patient TikToks. That is not science. That is marketing. That is misinformation.

You acknowledged the scale—622 million views on TikTok, a dataset larger than any trial in your field—and then dismissed it as "rare in doctor's offices." Of course it's rare in your offices: you don't measure it, you misdiagnose it, and patients no longer trust you enough to walk through your doors.

And when you confronted distrust, you did not ask whether patients had been harmed. You diagnosed the distrust itself—"cortico-phobia"—and called it pathology. You built scales to measure fear, but no registries to measure harm. You labeled patient resistance as irrational, while you ignored decades of published warnings and case series from your own colleagues around the world.

ISAD, this was not a scientific meeting. It was a plan to suppress TSW. The enemy was not eczema, but the patients who dared to tell the truth. And every word is on record.

The question is simple: when billions of testimonies are in plain sight, will you continue to retreat into your cave, or will you finally step into the light and study what is right in front of you?

Respectfully,

On behalf of patients whose stories are not misinformation, but evidence.

Source: International Society of Atopic Dermatitis (ISAD) Online Symposium, "The Cave of Misinformation," Spring 2025. Transcript and video available on YouTube.

My Anecdote Promise

In the preface, I told you there would be anecdotes in this book—stories you can hear and decide for yourself whether they are true. The following two letters are exactly that. Since I personally witnessed these encounters, these letters are written directly from me. Together, they illustrate two sides of dermatology's culture: open arrogance and quiet fear.

My Personal Letters to Dr. Curls and Dr. Anonymous

Exhibit F

Dear Dr. Curls,

I met you in Denver after I spoke at the American Academy of Dermatology meeting on the subject of topical steroid addiction and withdrawal. My husband and another member of our party—both of whom were in the same conversation when we spoke—were present. You approached me not with curiosity or collaboration, but with condescension. As the head of pediatric dermatology at a major university, you carried yourself like the sheriff of a sandbox I had no right to step into. And then, out of the blue, you opened the conversation like this:

"When I see a rash on a baby, I like to hit it hard with steroids."

I guess my presentation on the dangers of topical steroids had annoyed you. Those words are burned into my brain. They weren't careful. They weren't compassionate. They carried no humility, no hesitation, no concern for what might happen to those babies after the "hard" treatments you prescribed. They revealed your core philosophy: that faster, stronger, and more drug is always better—even for the most fragile patients in your care.

That is not medicine. That is domination. And it's the kind of thinking that has addicted an entire generation of children to topical steroids before they could even speak.

Dr. Curls, arrogance is not evidence. Bravado is not science. When you brag about "hitting it hard with steroids," you are not projecting confidence—you are broadcasting recklessness. You may wear a white coat, but to thousands of parents whose children now suffer through topical steroid withdrawal, your words echo more like a warning than advice.

Our children are not your proving ground. Their skin is not a canvas for pharmaceutical experimentation. What they need is restraint. What they deserve is protection.

And now—after learning about you in the last chapter—the world knows what else you bring into the exam room: over a million dollars in financial ties to the drug companies whose products you so aggressively promote. When you encourage fast, high-potency treatments while cashing checks from the same corporations that profit from prolonged dependency, it's not just a conflict of interest—it's a crisis of ethics.

What you call strength, we call harm. What you call decisive treatment, we call the start of an addiction cycle. And what you dismiss as fringe, we live as reality—scraped skin, sleepless nights, and doctors who refuse to listen.

You're not just part of the problem. You've become its mouthpiece. And you're getting paid handsomely to test new drugs on the very children you claim to protect. Our children deserved better than your arrogance.

Sincerely,

Kelly Palace

Exhibit G

Dear Dr. Anonymous,

During my research for this book, when I reached out to you, you told me you believe in TSA because you have seen it with your own eyes—in your own family. Your son suffered through it. And yet you begged me not to use your name.

Why? Because you are afraid. The son who went through TSW is now poised to enter medical school and wants to become a dermatologist. You fear that if the dermatology establishment learns the truth—

that you or your son acknowledge TSA—he will be ostracized. It will hurt his chances of ever becoming a dermatologist.

That is the level of control this profession exerts. Not only must patients stay silent, but even dermatologists who know the truth must whisper it in private, afraid of professional exile.

Your silence is as revealing as their denials. If telling the truth could ruin a young man's future in medicine, then dermatology has become less a field of science than a fortress of fear.

Sincerely,

Kelly Palace

‖‖

But there are exceptions to the voices of denial. A handful of dermatologists have broken ranks. Some of them deserve recognition here.

Exhibit H

Dear Supportive TSW Doctors,

We have not forgotten you. Beyond the pioneer researchers and whistleblowers already honored in these pages, there were others—the ones who looked us in the eye and said, *"I believe you."* The doctors who admitted what they had seen in their own patients, who treated us with caution, and who respected our suffering instead of dismissing it.

You are rare. And because of that, you are precious to us.

While others laughed, you listened. While others doubled down, you eased off the prescriptions and supported us through withdrawal. While others told us it was "all in our heads," you treated us as human beings, not medical inconveniences.

To be believed, to be respected, to be guided gently instead of gaslit and harmed—these things saved us. Not the creams. Not the protocols. You.

We wish there were more of you. We wish your courage was the rule instead of the exception. We wish your compassion wasn't so rare that we remember every one of your names years later.

From the depths of our pain, we thank you. And we carry the hope that someday, you won't be the outliers—you will be the standard.

The evidence speaks for itself. From the podium to the podcast, from the Instagram feed to the university clinic, the message has been consistent: deny, minimize, rebrand, intimidate, overprescribe. Whether wrapped in jokes, legal disclaimers, arrogance, or outright bullying, the result is the same—patients left unheard, untreated, and unseen. These six letters are not just stories. They are a map of how denial is maintained, how arrogance is rewarded, and how fear keeps even the truth-tellers silent. This is what happens when a profession builds a fortress to protect itself instead of protecting the people it was meant to serve.

In a field so often defined by deniers, the most valuable and appreciated doctors are those who can listen, learn, and change their minds. Dr. Peter Lio is one of them.

Exhibit I

Dear Newer TSW Expert Dr. Peter Lio,

You may remember from *Presence and Prevalence* that we included your voice as one of the few dermatologists willing to acknowledge topical steroid withdrawal (TSW) openly and respectfully. In a field where so many minimize, dismiss, or mock, your willingness to stand on a stage at the 2025 *Revolutionizing Atopic Dermatitis (RAD) Conference* and treat TSW as real was a gift to patients who have spent decades being silenced.

You explained not only that you see TSW, but why your colleagues may struggle to accept it. That they may feel threatened or usurped because this isn't the way most patients show up. You said you think it might be a weird reaction from fellow doctors because it's backwards when a patient says, "I think I have TSW". Doctors usually diagnose and not the patients.

That honesty matters. You didn't dismiss patients for daring to bring you a name for their condition. You didn't call them "phobic." You acknowledged both the clinical pattern and the emotional dynamics at play—and in doing so, you showed your peers a better way forward.

For patients like us, after years of being told "this condition does not exist," your words were a breath of oxygen. You gave us not only recognition, but an explanation for the wall we so often hit in exam rooms. You reminded us that our voices aren't the threat; they are part of the evidence.

Thank you for being willing to change your mind. Thank you for being willing to listen. And thank you for showing your colleagues that humility in medicine is not weakness—it's strength.

Dr. Lio proves something critical: doctors can change their minds. They can listen, learn, and even admit that patients sometimes see what medicine has overlooked. But if one doctor can do this, why not more? And if the evidence is mounting, why does the denial remain so entrenched? The answer lies beyond individual exam rooms.

The Bigger Fortress

The doctors were only the first line of denial. Behind them stand bigger forces—agencies and corporations with even more at stake. If dermatologists mocked, minimized, or silenced us, it was because the system they serve created, cultivated and fed into the massive disconnect. In the US, the FDA, the very agency meant to protect patients, turned its gaze away and has refused to take responsibility, touting that the outcome of TSW was a "practice of medicine" problem, not theirs. Big Pharma—the multi-billion-dollar machine that makes and markets the drugs—fueled the silence with money, influence, and intimidation. And the American Academy of Dermatology (AAD), whose clinical care guidelines serve as the gold standard for all skin conditions, has continually refused to take the concerns of patients seriously.

The final letter is to the AAD.

Exhibit J

Dear American Academy of Dermatology,

If this were a courtroom, you would be the expert witness on the stand. You've sworn an oath to protect patients, to tell the truth. But I must ask: how can you stand so steadfast when the ground beneath you is this shaky?

You tell patients—and the doctors you train—that topical steroids are safe. You tell the public that topical steroid withdrawal is nothing more than uncontrolled eczema. But where is your proof? Not claims. Not consensus statements. Not reassurances based on "decades of use." Real proof.

An attorney would say: **I demand you show the evidence.**

- **Show us the long-term safety data on infants and children treated continuously or repeatedly with topical steroids over months and years. Where are those studies?**

- Show us the prospective research proving these drugs do not cause dependence or withdrawal—even though patient reports and published case series say otherwise.

- Show us the comparative evidence that withdrawal is indistinguishable from eczema, when entire cohorts of patients describe new, distinct patterns of burning, oozing, spreading rashes that never existed before treatment.

- Show us the guidelines and disclosures where you warned patients that withdrawal was even a possibility. Where is the informed consent?

If you cannot produce this evidence, then your position is not science. It is dogma. It is opinion propped up by habit, industry influence, and fear of liability.

Doctors look to you for guidance. Patients depend on you for truth. But right now, your guidance is silence, and your truth is denial.

So the question is simple: will you provide updated proof—not 70-year-old proof, not from consensus committees, but from real, current, independent, long-term studies—that topical steroids are safe and that topical steroid withdrawal is merely "eczema"? Or will you continue to stand steadfast on shaky ground?

Respectfully,

On behalf of patients who deserve more than reassurances.

—————————————————————————————

If this chapter exposes the arrogance and fear inside dermatology, the next one reveals the real fortress: the regulators, corporations, doctor organizations and those who keep a broken system running on the backs of people who are sick and addicted to medications that are a bandaid, not a cure. The power players.

—————————————————————————————

CHAPTER FIFTEEN

THE FORTRESS: FDA AND BIG PHARMA

IN THE LAST CHAPTER, WE SAW HOW dermatologists themselves act as soldiers in the resistance, and how the final courtroom-style letter to the American Academy of Dermatology exposed that organization as a key part of the fortress. The AAD is not just part of the fortress; it is the barracks inside the wall, churning out soldiers armed with outdated dogma and shielded by industry ties. It keeps the ranks full, the guidelines rigid, and the denial intact—all while marching in lockstep with pharma and the FDA.

On my phone one recent morning, the FDA was in the headlines again: this time, warning Americans that certain foam sunscreens weren't properly approved and might not protect us.[1] Within hours, it was national news. That's the power of three letters—FDA. When they speak, people listen.

Over the years, the agency has issued dozens of similar warnings—from contaminated eye drops to mislabeled supplements to itching after stopping an antihistamine.[2] But here's what they've never done: issue a single black-box warning against any topical steroid.[3] Not even a basic label warning patients that using these creams can cause addiction and withdrawal. Silence.

And that silence matters. Because unlike the National Eczema Association or the American Academy of Dermatology—the FDA could stop this entire chain of harm tomorrow. If they said no more topical steroids or warned of their potential for damage, doctors either couldn't prescribe them or would think twice about it. Period.

The FDA's Inaction

There was no better person to interview for this section than ITSAN's current President, Kelly Barta. For years, she has been knocking on the FDA's door, armed with hundreds of patient reports and a mountain of evidence. What she encountered wasn't just silence. It was something worse—acknowledgment without action.

"They basically said, we know about this. So do medical providers. The doctors are just not telling their patients. This is a problem within the practice of medicine."

That one line captures everything wrong with the FDA's position on topical steroid withdrawal. They admit they know, yet push responsibility onto doctors who themselves don't even recognize the condition. The patients are left trapped in a cycle where no one is accountable.

Kelly wasn't alone in raising alarms. While serving as ITSAN president, she personally gathered 500 patient reports that had been submitted through the FDA's own Adverse-Event Reporting System (AERS). The FDA's reply was chilling.

"I had 500 people from our group confirm they reported to the FDA. And when we asked about a threshold signalling the need to take action, the Deputy Director of Safety for the FDA's Center for Drug Evaluation and Research (CDER) told us: 'There is no threshold. We already know about it. You can tell your people they don't need to report—because we already know about these outcomes. This issue is not our problem.'"

This is whistleblowing 101: patients followed the rules, did what the agency asks, and were told the rules don't matter.

When Kelly pressed harder, she unearthed something that reads like a scene out of *The Insider*. She found a 2007 FDA guidance document on the agency's website—one in which they promised to be "the primary source of drug safety information" for doctors and patients, to proactively warn the public whenever harms were discovered. When she cited it back to FDA officials in a meeting, the document mysteriously vanished from their website.[4]

This wasn't just denial. It felt like erasure.

Kelly's experience echoed a tragic precedent. She recalls watching the final episode of *Dopesick* **the night before her follow-up FDA meeting. The show laid bare how, in the opioid crisis, regulators failed to act decisively even when presented with staggering evidence of harm.**

"Before that meeting, I watched the last episode of *Dopesick*. I was glad I did, because it prepared me. The show made clear how the FDA didn't take responsibility in the opioid epidemic—even after being shown 400 autopsy reports. They still wouldn't act. After watching how things played out in that scenario, I wasn't surprised by the response we were given, but still was deeply discouraged and truly angered that they resisted taking responsibility in the case of TSW too."

The pattern is clear. Semmelweis warned about handwashing and was mocked. Barry Marshall swallowed *H. pylori* and was ridiculed. Flint's children drank lead-tainted water while officials reassured parents it was safe. Tobacco companies told us cigarettes were harmless for decades. Each time, history revealed the same arc: denial, delay, deflection—until the human toll was undeniable. TSW sits on that same continuum, and the FDA's current stance makes the outcome predictable.

And the hypocrisy is galling. Just last year, the FDA issued a public health advisory for Zyrtec withdrawal itching—warning consumers that stopping the antihistamine could trigger rebound symptoms.[6] Yet for topical steroids—a class of drugs that can devastate lives for years—nothing.

"They issued a public health advisory for Zyrtec withdrawal itching—but won't do the same for topical steroids destroying people's lives."

The FDA is not neutral here. Their silence is not accidental. It protects an industry worth billions and a terribly broken system. And when you see how easily a warning is issued for an antihistamine, while thousands of steroid-injured patients are told their suffering is "the practice of medicine," you begin to understand that the problem isn't ignorance. It's alignment coupled with slow-as-molasses bureaucracy.

Kelly Barta's testimony is a case study in futility: patients did everything by the book, the FDA admitted awareness, documents disappeared, warnings never came, and communications stayed faceless, nameless, and unaccountable.

Unlike the UK equivalent of the FDA—the MHRA (Medicines and Healthcare products Regulatory Agency)—which actually responded to patient concerns and partnered with dermatology associations, that kind of collaboration has never happened in the United States. In the U.S., patient voices have been sidelined, and the FDA has yet to mandate a single warning about TSW on steroid packaging.

From here, the narrative widens. Because the FDA does not exist in isolation. Its silence is symbiotic with the pharmaceutical companies who write the checks, fund the studies, and invent new formulations to keep profits flowing.

Enter Big Pharma

If the FDA is the watchdog that won't bite, it's because the watchdog is being fed by the very hands it's supposed to guard against. By 2024, nearly half of the FDA's $7.2 billion budget—about $3.3 billion—came not from taxpayers but from industry user fees.[7] In its drug review division, the dependency was even starker: 77% of funding came directly from pharmaceutical companies.[8]

Pharma pays to be regulated.

And the money at stake is staggering. The global topical corticosteroids market—the category that includes creams, ointments, and foams—was valued at nearly $5 billion in 2021, with projections to climb to $8–18 billion by 2030.[9] These aren't just creams and ointments; they are billion-dollar revenue streams disguised as standard care.

That financial tie colors everything. It creates an incentive structure where speed and volume of drug approvals matter far more than long-term safety—or inconvenient truths like withdrawal syndromes. A slow approval or a public health advisory that rattles confidence isn't just bad for Pharma's profits. It starves the FDA's own revenue stream.

And Pharma knows how to play the game. When a branded drug approaches the cliff of generic competition, "innovation" often doesn't mean a safer or more effective treatment. Instead, it means a new formulation: a cream becomes an ointment, and an ointment becomes a foam. A label tweak, a new delivery system, and suddenly the "same drug" is reborn as a higher-priced branded product.[10]

I saw it firsthand during my years as a Pfizer drug rep, more formally known as a pharmaceutical sales rep. One afternoon, I was standing in the hallway outside a busy physician's office, waiting for my turn with the doctor. The corridor smelled faintly of alcohol wipes and coffee. Another pharma company's representative was already detailing the doctor, and I was next in line to speak with her.

That's when I overheard what she was saying. Her tone was conspiratorial, almost cheerful: "I know patients love the steroid creams," she told him, "but we're launching a foam. Same drug, just a different formulation."

The honesty of it was surprising—an admission that nothing was really new. No breakthrough, no safer alternative, just a new wrapper for an old product. This was the playbook: swap out a vehicle, slap on a new label, extend the patent life, and reopen a profitable revenue stream.[10]

That moment stuck with me. Years later, sitting in a dermatologist's office as a patient, I was offered a foam formulation as an alternative to the steroid creams they usually prescribed. I remember thinking: Aha. I've seen this trick before.

That convergence—of my past as a rep and my future as a patient—was eye-opening. It revealed how the industry's games weren't abstract. They landed in my own chart, on my own skin.

Dependency Generates Dollars

Because that's the larger truth: Pharma thrives not on curing disease, but on reformulating dependence. And the FDA, financially entangled with the very industry it's supposed to regulate, has no incentive to disrupt this pipeline.

The result is systemic:

- Patients cycle endlessly through products that are, in essence, the same addictive drug in different bottles.
- Doctors keep prescribing updated products.
- Pharma keeps profiting.
- The FDA keeps collecting fees—and stays silent.

And the epidemic of dependence and withdrawal grinds on, unchecked.

Threading FDA + Pharma Together

The FDA does not exist in isolation. It is entwined with the very industry it is meant to police. Nearly half of its operating budget now comes from industry user fees,[11] and in drug review the dependence runs as high as 70–77%.[12] This means the companies under FDA scrutiny are also the ones footing its bills. A watchdog that eats from the same hand it's supposed to bite will never bite very hard.

The relationship is symbiotic. Pharma gains a regulator incentivized to move drugs quickly through the pipeline. The FDA gains a steady revenue stream to keep its operations afloat. Both sides are served. Only patients are left unprotected.

History shows how this dynamic can play out. In the 1980s, Bayer's Cutter Laboratories sold clotting factor products contaminated with HIV. After the company introduced a safer, heat-treated version for the U.S. market, it continued shipping the older, unsafe batches overseas. When the issue surfaced, the FDA ordered Cutter to stop the practice quietly—but chose not to alert Congress, physicians, or the public.[13] The oversight agency acted not as a whistleblower, but as a shield for industry.

The parallels are hard to ignore. As with contaminated clotting factors, topical steroids continue to circulate in the market without meaningful warning. Both cases reveal the same pattern: when patient safety collides with corporate profits and regulatory dependence, silence wins.

And this silence is not neutral. It is alignment. The FDA and Pharma move in tandem—not adversaries, but bedfellows. The agency's authority gives the appearance of protection; Pharma's dollars keep the machine running. Together, they ensure the cycle of prescribing, dependence, and reformulation continues unchecked.

Closing the Circle

If the FDA wanted to stop this epidemic, it could tomorrow. With a single black-box warning, or a public health advisory, the cascade of overprescribing would grind to a halt. Dermatologists would be forced to pause, patients would be alerted, and Pharma's marketing carousel of creams, ointments, and foams would lose momentum.[15]

But that has not happened. And the reason is no longer mysterious. **The FDA and Pharma are not merely in dialogue—they are in alignment.** The regulator survives on the industry's dollars; the industry thrives on the regulator's silence. It is a closed system that perpetuates dependence by design.

Patients, meanwhile, are left as collateral damage—their lives frayed, their health dismissed, their warnings ignored. It is a system that protects itself before it protects the public.

When those in power failed, leaders within the patient movement became the only safeguard against silence.

References

1. FDA Warning Letter re: unapproved foam sunscreens (Aug. 6, 2025). [FDA.gov]

2. FDA Drug Safety Communications; *The Medical Letter,* "Cetirizine Withdrawal Itching," May 2025.

3. FDA/DailyMed drug labels for clobetasol foam (Impeklo), triamcinolone, betamethasone (no boxed warning).

4. FDA, *Guidance for Industry: Communicating Drug Safety Information,* 2007 (archived version).

5. *Dopesick* (Hulu series), Episode 8, 2021; dramatization of FDA inaction during opioid epidemic.

6. FDA Drug Safety Communication, Cetirizine withdrawal itch, May 2025.

7. FDA, *At a Glance: FY 2024,* October 2024.

8. FDA, FY 2024 PDUFA Financial Report, Table 11, p. 6.

9. Spherical Insights, *Topical Corticosteroids Market Report*, 2022; DataIntelo, *Topical Steroids Market Forecast*, 2023.

10. FDA NDA Approval, OLUX Foam (clobetasol propionate), 2000; Connetics SEC Filing, OLUX-E, 2007.

11. FDA, *At a Glance: FY 2024*, October 2024. https://www.fda.gov/media/182749/download

12. FDA, FY 2024 PDUFA Financial Report, Table 11, p. 6. https://www.fda.gov/media/184951/download

13. *New York Times*, "2 Paths of Bayer Drug in 80's: Riskier Type Went Overseas," May 22, 2003; *The Guardian*, "Bayer Sold HIV-Contaminated Blood Products," May 23, 2003.

14. FDA, *Boxed Warnings Overview*, 2024 (examples of drugs where FDA has acted rapidly to warn the public).

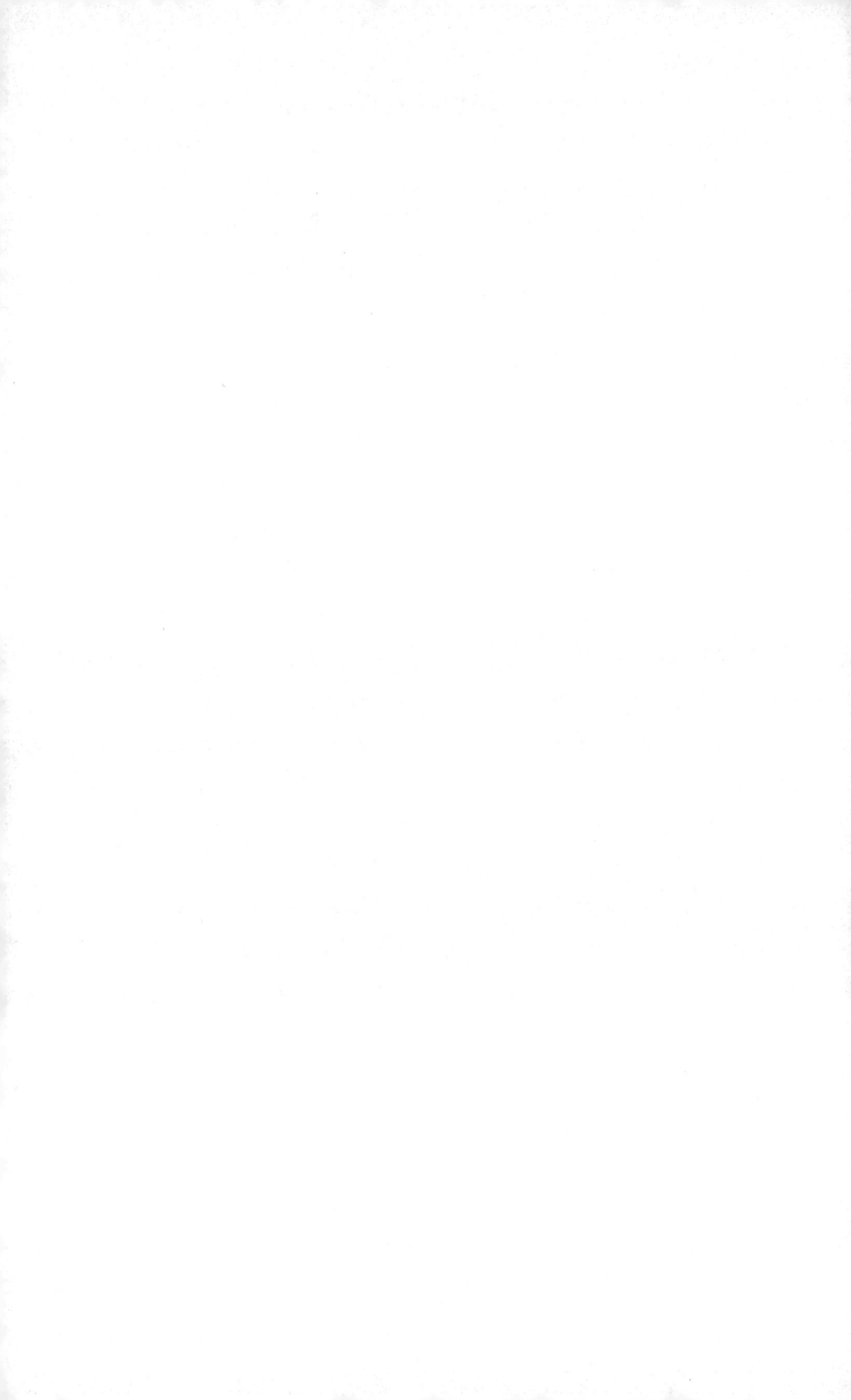

PART VI

THE ADVOCATES AND ACTIVISTS

CHAPTER SIXTEEN

WHY WE FIGHT

IN CENTRAL SCOTLAND, THE LAUGHTER of three children drifts down the hallway of a modest home. Lilly is seven, Harley five, and little Robyn just four—all bursting with the energy of childhood, chasing one another in the living room, squealing in delight. Their father, Tom Drysdale, listens from the next room. He wants to join them. More than anything, he wants to scoop them up, wrestle, play, be the kind of active, rough-and-tumble dad he once was. But his body won't let him.

Tom is in the middle of another period of skin hell. His body is raw, burning, stretched so tight it splits if he laughs too hard. A simple burst of joy can trigger a wave of hives, a storm of itch that rips through him like fire. He cannot sweat. He cannot get overheated. Even the lightest touch of water feels like acid. To play with his children would mean agony, hours of recovery, maybe days. So he stays where he is—close enough to hear their laughter, far enough to keep from breaking.

This is the theft that topical steroid withdrawal commits. It doesn't just wound the body; it steals moments, memories, milestones. For Tom, it has stolen piggyback rides, games of chase, bedtime baths. It has turned him into a spectator of his own children's childhoods. "I'm a shadow of the person I was," he says. And when he says it, he isn't only mourning his skin—he's mourning the father he longs to be.

Yet even in this brokenness, Tom has chosen to fight. Not because he is whole, but because he isn't. Not because he has time or energy to spare, but because he has lost too much already. His story is not unique. It is the story of every patient-volunteer who builds this movement on a body that is itself in ruins.

Tom in Action

It was 2021 during one of those nights—3 a.m., standing in his kitchen after yet another itch attack, too raw to sleep, too restless to sit—that Tom opened his laptop in search of answers to help ease his suffering. What he found was ITSAN. He didn't just see it as a patient seeking comfort; he saw it through another lens. With a background in branding and storytelling, Tom could see what the charity was missing—and what it could become. Even in the middle of his pain, a thought formed: *maybe I can help.*

Tom isn't just surviving TSW—he's redesigning the way the world sees it. Before his body broke down, he spent a decade in London's creative industry, working in brand activation, as an Art Director and Designer. He knows how to take an idea and give it shape, how to craft a message that cuts through noise, how to rally strangers around a shared story. When he found ITSAN, he didn't just see a small nonprofit—he saw a movement without a platform to fight from.

What struck him was the gap. The medical diplomacy mattered, yes—but the story wasn't being told in a way that captured the raw urgency patients lived with every day. Tom saw a community that needed not only information, but identity. He envisioned a digital heartbeat for the movement: **the TSW Action Hub.**

True to the spirit of ITSAN, Tom's designs for the Action Hub were made real through the talents of a web developer whose loved one developed TSW, spurring him to reach out and volunteer. Likewise, ITSAN board members Kelly Barta, Nick Geller, Sarat Pothuri, and Natalie Lawton pulled together to help get the initiative off the ground.

"The Action Hub isn't about one creative individual's ideas," Tom said. "It takes a shared vision and a whole team pulling together to make it happen. That's what makes it powerful. It's really important to point out that it was—and truly is—a collaborative process."

The Hub is not a website for browsing. It is a rallying point. **A place where patients can turn pain into purpose.** On it, people can:

- Join the world's first TSW patient registry to help prove TSW is real
- Advocate for state-level recognition to put TSW on the map
- Expose the truth about TSW by sharing our awareness page
- Report their condition to official bodies to help build pressure
- Sign our petition to add weight to every campaign we run
- Download resources to educate their doctor about TSW
- Find support to alert the press and share their own story
- Fundraise and donate to fuel our mission, supporting the TSW community

At the heart of the Hub is a message Tom helped shape: **Protect. Prove. Prevent.**

- **Protect** those who are suffering right now.
- **Prove** the harm through data, stories, and undeniable evidence.
- **Prevent** this crisis from destroying more lives in the future.

This is branding at its best—simple, memorable, repeatable. It gives patients language they can hold onto in the storm. It turns a fragile network of hurting people into a cause with structure and clarity.

And yet, Tom hasn't stopped here. He has created a toolkit of brand communications that give the TSW community a vehicle to focus their frustration into meaningful action; and help unaware audiences grasp the severity and scale of the TSW crisis. Even housebound, he has found purpose amidst the pain. And he took his commitment one step further, joining ITSAN's board of directors in 2025.

But perhaps his most powerful contribution is not visual at all. It's spoken. At ITSAN's request, Tom asked the community to name what they had lost to TSW—birthdays, jobs, relationships, confidence, health. He gathered those fragments and forged them into a collective cry. The result was a poem—equal parts lament and battle hymn.

Why I Fight: A Rallying Cry from the TSW Community

For the nights I woke bleeding, alone in my bed,
For the tears on my pillow, the fear in my head.
For the body torn open, the pain without peace,
For the itch that consumed me, no hope of release.

For the skin that would split when I smiled or spoke,
For the months I just lay there, trying to cope.
For the food I feared and the water that stung,
For the dreams that were stolen before they'd begun.

For the moments I missed, when I couldn't be near,
For the warmth that was lost with those I hold dear.
For the clothes that clung to the weeping and red,
For the mirror I covered, the words left unsaid.

For the friends who stopped calling, the stares on the street,
For the bonds that were shattered, too fragile to keep.
For the doctors who shrugged and turned me away,
For the prayers that I whispered at break of each day.

For the birthdays alone and the silence so deep,
For the wounds I still carry, too painful to speak.
For the times I begged my own heart to stop,
For the mornings I rose—just to fall, then to drop.

For the souls still trapped in this hot, burning flame,
For the trauma inflicted, medication to blame.
For the voices unheard, the truth pushed aside,
For the harm that goes on—by "experts", denied.

For the ones yet to suffer this cruel, hellish fate,
For the chance to protect them before it's too late.
For the right to be heard, to be seen, to feel whole—
I fight to reclaim the life steroids stole.

This is not just Tom's voice. It is the voice of thousands who suffer in silence. His words, line by line, are being filmed and read by patients around the globe. Together they form a chorus—fragile, scarred, defiant.

This is why we fight.

Every Volunteer's Story

Tom's story is extraordinary. But it is also ordinary in this movement. For every communication he creates, for every line of poetry he crafts, there are hundreds of other patients and parents giving in quieter ways—an email answered, a forum post written in the middle of the night, a fundraiser organized between flare-ups, a board meeting attended from a hospital bed.

This is what makes ITSAN unique. It is not powered by polished professionals with unlimited stamina. It is built on suffering bodies—people who are themselves sick, depleted, and sometimes barely hanging on. No one here can give all the time. People disappear for weeks or months during hard times, then come back when they can. Leadership shifts not only because of transitions, but because illness forces it. The rhythm of our advocacy follows the rhythm of our pain.

And yet, the miracle is that the work continues. Even in the midst of brokenness, a mosaic of small contributions keeps adding up: a mother in Nevada writing to her senator, a patient in India organizing awareness at her clinic, a caregiver in Canada posting another story to social media. One person drops the torch; another picks it up. No one carries it alone.

Tom's Action Hub vision captures this reality: that the fight against TSW is both international and deeply personal, fueled by a global chorus of hurting people who still choose to act. He is not the exception. He is the example.

Scratch That: **The UK's Advocate Voice**

Back in the *Presence and Prevalence* chapter, I promised we would circle back to the UK—and the work happening there. The UK is the only country besides the United States with a formal organization dedicated to advocating for Topical Steroid Withdrawal (TSW) awareness and recognition. That organization is *Scratch That*.

Founded as a patient-led movement, *Scratch That* became a lifeline for sufferers across Britain. Their mission has always been clear: to raise awareness of TSW, to validate the suffering of patients, and to push for recognition in both medical and regulatory systems. Their messaging is both bold and healing: TSW is not your fault. TSW is not "just severe eczema." And topical steroid addiction is not a psychological dependence. By separating myth from truth, *Scratch That* has given the UK community not only validation, but a banner to rally under.

What makes *Scratch That* especially powerful is that they don't just tell stories—they organize. They provide education about the long, grueling recovery process, offer practical resources like their *MP Letter Guide* for contacting Members of Parliament, and keep pressure on the medical establishment to acknowledge the reality of this condition. They've turned patient pain into civic action.

And that action worked. Perhaps their biggest victory so far came when the UK's Medicines and Healthcare products Regulatory Agency (MHRA) formally acknowledged TSW in 2021. The MHRA is the British equivalent of the U.S. FDA, overseeing drug safety. After years of denial, the agency mandated that warnings about TSW must appear in both the Summary of Product Characteristics (SmPC) for prescribers and the Patient Information Leaflets (PILs) that go into every box of topical steroid sold in the UK. This wasn't a small foot-note—it was a seismic shift. For the first time, TSW was enshrined in official drug labeling.

Scratch That's advocacy also helped push the broader conversation into the mainstream medical community. The National Eczema So-ciety (NES), together with the British Association of Dermatologists (BAD) and nursing groups, issued joint position statements on TSW. While those statements often tried to soften or reframe the issue, the fact remains: patient voices, amplified by *Scratch That*, led to the UK's largest dermatology organizations publicly acknowledging what had long been dismissed as anecdote.

In advocacy terms, this was no small feat. TSW moved from in-ternet forums and whispered stories to official medical documents and professional statements. Patients could now point to the very leaflet in their hands and say: *"Look. It's real. It's written here."* That legitimacy is priceless—and it was won through years of patient-led persistence.

The lesson for advocates is clear: change doesn't come from si-lence. *Scratch That* shows what's possible when patient communities organize, speak with clarity, and refuse to be brushed aside. They prove that even in the face of entrenched denial, grassroots activism can reshape the narrative, shift medical language, and put new warnings into the hands of every family opening a tube of cream.

As a call back to our FDA chapter: unlike the FDA, the UK equivalent—the MHRA—actually responded to patient concerns and partnered with dermatology associations. That kind of collaboration has *never* happened in the United States. In the U.S., patient voices have been sidelined, and the FDA has yet to mandate a single warning about TSW on steroid packaging. The UK broke that mold.

The UK's Activist Voice

The UK also has a group of activists who have staged the "TSW March in March" for the past four years. This year's gathering, held on March 29th in Archbishop's Park, London, drew more than 100 people carrying signs, speaking through megaphones, and sharing raw, emotional testimonials. The organizers didn't hold back in announcing the event on Instagram, calling TSW *"Seriously, Traumatic, Excruciating, Ravaging, Overpowering, Invasive, Devastating... Shit."* Among my favorite images from the march was a sign that read: *"Doctors, Flake Off!"*—a stinging bit of wordplay that hit especially hard because one of the most relentless symptoms of TSW is the incessant flaking of skin.

I have so much love and respect for these activists. When writing this section, I tried, but was unable to reach the organizers of this movement. But hats off to their courage, their creativity, their refusal to be silenced—it's the heartbeat of this movement. All information I've included here is available online. If I weren't a journalist and the co-founder of ITSAN, I would absolutely be one of them, marching with a sign in one hand and a megaphone in the other. In many ways, I already am. The fire they carry is the same fire that fuels me—and I'm just as angry. I've simply had to channel my outrage through words, interviews, and organizational leadership. But make no mistake: their voices and mine are part of the same chorus, demanding recognition, justice, and healing. I'm so glad they are part of this fight. We need every voice. We need every fighter. We need them all.

That brings us to an important distinction in every movement— the difference between *advocates* and *activists*. Both are vital, and both shape the TSW fight.

Advocates vs. Activists: Two Sides of the Same Fight

At first glance, the words *advocate* and *activist* sound interchangeable. Both describe people who care deeply about a cause and want to see change. But there's a definite difference in tone and approach. In the social media revolution chapter we met mostly activists. Patient organizations are usually more like advocates.

Advocates are often the bridge builders. They focus on raising awareness, providing education, and influencing decision-makers through dialogue. An advocate works within systems—meeting with lawmakers, presenting research to medical bodies, or creating resources for patients and families. Advocacy tends to sound measured, professional, and diplomatic. It's about being the steady, reasoned voice that convinces others to take a closer look.

Activists, by contrast, are the fire-starters. They're the ones willing to march, protest, organize campaigns, and make noise that can't be ignored. Activism is about urgency, disruption, and passion—forcing those in power to confront what they would rather avoid. Activists shift public opinion, break through apathy, and push movements forward when polite appeals aren't enough.

Both roles are essential. Advocacy without activism risks being ignored. Activism without advocacy risks being dismissed. Together, they create the one-two punch that makes change possible. In the TSW movement, we have needed both: **advocates** who craft letters to regulators, meet with politicians, and publish careful research, and **activists** who light up social media, share raw photos, and demand accountability. One steadies the hand. The other lights the fire.

Young Oliver Feels Heard

In the UK, advocacy isn't only happening online, in public marches or regulatory offices—it's happening in community halls, parks, and coffee shops, too. One of the brightest new efforts is **TSW Together**, founded in 2025 by **Chloe Tatton**, a 25-year-old from Cheshire who has lived through TSW herself. Prescribed her first steroid cream at three months old, Chloe used steroids on and off for nearly 24 years under the guidance of doctors. By her early twenties, her skin showed the unmistakable signs of topical steroid addiction, though she was told it was just "severe eczema." It wasn't until she did her own research and stopped using steroids altogether that she went into full-blown TSW—what she describes as the most horrific and challenging experience of her life.

Born out of that suffering, Chloe founded **TSW Together** in April 2025 with a simple truth: withdrawal is incredibly isolating, and no one should have to go through it alone. What started as an online presence on TikTok and Instagram, where she documented her skin journey, became a real-world support hub. TSW Together now hosts **in-person events** for the TSW community, bringing patients, care-givers, and allies together in safe, uplifting spaces. Their mission is to build friendship, champion skin confidence, and raise awareness through education and storytelling.

At their first event in Manchester in June 2025, **Chloe remembers a 14-year-old boy named Oliver,** who had been in TSW since he was 8, telling her: *"For the first time, I've been able to get how this has affected me off my chest, because I'm surrounded by people who truly get it. It feels like a family."* That moment, Chloe says, solidified her purpose: turning pain into connection, and connection into healing.

TSW Together is still small, but it's growing—with dreams of expanding across the UK and, one day, internationally. Chloe hopes not just to build community but also to sit on panels with dermatologists, sharing the lived reality of TSW to a profession that has long denied it. Her work embodies the bridge between **advocacy and activism**: not loud protest, not policy briefs, but something equally radical—giving people a place to belong.

From why we fight to what we're fighting for, the story now turns to the future.

CHAPTER SEVENTEEN
PAIN INTO POWER

||||||||||||||||||||||||||||||||||||||||||||||||||||||||||||||||||||||||||||||||||||||||||||||||||||||||||||||||||||||||||||||||||||||||||

HELL HATH NO FURY LIKE A WOMAN scorned, or a TSW survivor. This chapter is about torchbearers. They weren't polished spokespeople or career advocates—they were ordinary people pushed into extraordinary roles. They were women whose own skin was breaking, who still found the strength to organize, to comfort, to build something larger than themselves. Their leadership was born not of privilege, but of necessity.

Many voices helped carry this movement—men and women, parents and patients, caregivers and allies. But when it came to steering the organization of ITSAN itself, the presidency fell, time after time, to women in the thick of their own withdrawal. They led not because they had the strength to spare, but because the fight demanded it.

Leadership in a patient–led movement is not a title—it's a torch carried through exhaustion, illness, and resistance. For ITSAN, that torch has passed through the hands of four women who each knew the fight from the inside out. We came to this role not from political campaigns or corporate ladders, but from hospital beds, doctor's offices, and the long nights of wondering if anyone would ever believe us. Each president inherited a different landscape—sometimes scorched earth, sometimes fertile ground—but the mission never changed: to give TSW sufferers a voice, a name, and a chance at justice. This chapter tells our story in reverse, beginning with today's battles and working back to the organization's first days. Four women. Four seasons of leadership. One relentless cause.

We begin with the woman holding the torch today—a leader whose path to the podium began in the ashes of personal loss and the depths of TSW's grip.

After twenty-one years of marriage, Kelly Barta's life was coming apart at the seams. She and her husband had once been fiercely in love—raising two children, building a home filled with ordinary joys—but now, as with so many others in the TSW community, the shadow of separation on multiple levels had led to a decision of divorce. Her husband, once her constant caretaker and champion, was being crushed under the strain of her prolonged illness and had reached a breaking point. What began as love-driven care had evolved into duty, and that duty had turned into a quiet bitterness. Her health was still recovering from the years-long storm of TSW and her heart was torn in two from the dissolution of her marriage. And yet, at the very moment when most people would retreat, Kelly was about to step into the most public, demanding role of her life.

She had served on ITSAN's board since 2016, propelled by a sense of calling that felt bigger than her own circumstances. In April 2018, she was elected president of the only nonprofit in the world solely dedicated to TSW awareness and advocacy. Since then, she has made—and continues to make—some of the most important gains in the fight for TSW protection, both in proving the harm and preventing it.

Kelly Barta—Survivor to Strategist

When Kelly Barta takes the podium at national or international events, and she often does, she carries the weight of lived experience and the authority of a seasoned advocate. Her calm, graceful bearing—paired with a quiet but unmistakable passion—draws people in and makes them listen. She served as President of ITSAN from April 2018 to October 2019, and again from November 2024 to today, where she is ITSAN's current president. In the years between her presidencies, while still heavily involved in ITSAN's work, she built influential relationships and amassed the kind of hard-won knowledge that positioned her to return with the power to change the entire conversation about TSW.

Her leadership portfolio beyond ITSAN includes working with the National Eczema Association, the Allergy & Asthma Network, and leading the Coalition of Skin Diseases (CSD), where she became president in 2020, transitioned to full-time at CSD in 2022, and continued through the summer of 2025. She currently serves on the American Academy of Dermatology's Patient Advocacy Task Force, the Atopic Eczema Advisory Council for Global Skin, and the FDA/CTTI's Patient Engagement Collaborative.

Her appointments to advisory councils within historically resistant organizations aren't signs of their transformation so much as proof of her persistence. Kelly's credibility, built on both survival and strategy, has opened doors in places that once dismissed TSW outright. She enters these rooms not because the institutions have fully embraced the truth, but because she has continued to press forward in advocacy, embracing opportunities to build relationship and continue telling the TSW story until it can no longer be ignored.

In 2022, she penned her memoir, *To Eczema, with Love*, and was featured in the *Epoch Times* late 2024 and the *New York Post* in 2025, sharing her TSW story—cementing her place as one of the most compelling and courageous voices for TSW awareness today.

Over a decade into the TSW fight, her voice has reached regulators, policymakers, medical conferences, and legislative chambers—always carrying the same message: TSW is real, it's devastating, and it must be addressed.

A Life in Eczema's Grip

Kelly's skin story began in childhood. As a preteen, she was prescribed topical steroids—the standard treatment for eczema. Over the decades, her skin demanded stronger prescriptions until she was using one of the highest-potency creams on the market: betamethasone dipropionate.

Life with eczema was a constant negotiation. Rain could bring a rash. So could gardening, intimacy, or the linens at a hotel. She developed food and environmental allergies, and with each year, her world grew smaller.

Her doctors dismissed her questions about whether certain foods or substances could be making her skin react. "Eczema is hereditary," they told her. "You'll drive yourself crazy looking for triggers. You just need to accept the fact that you'll need to use a steroid cream for the rest of your life."

The Moment of Doubt

The first crack in that confidence came from an unexpected place: the pharmacy counter. A new technician glanced at her prescription, saw the drug's potency, and asked how long she'd been on it. When Kelly answered, "About ten years," the tech's startled expression said more than words. She warned Kelly to be cautious. It was the first time a medical professional had ever voiced concern. That tiny moment of honesty sent Kelly digging for answers.

Kelly's Descent

She began weaning herself off steroids, hoping to reduce her allergies. Two days after stopping completely, the burning began—paired with a bone-deep itching so fierce it made her want to claw off her skin. Over the next three weeks, the red patches of burning skin, which had erupted first on her arms and neck, spread to cover her entire body.

Over the next 18 months, Kelly's world collapsed into a prison of her bed and the bathtub. The tub was the only place that dulled the agony, so she lived between the two. Her skin oozed, shed in sheets, and smelled foul from the constant exudate. Her hair fell out. She developed a cataract that required surgery. Even reaching for the TV remote was a calculated risk to avoid pain.

"This was not eczema," she says. "This was unregulated body temperature, nerve zingers, intense itching, ooze, anxiety, insomnia and weight loss. It was the feeling of being scalded from head to toe."

She couldn't work. She couldn't care for her two boys. Her 21-year marriage ended. She lost years she will never get back.

The Virus That Nearly Ended Her Life

Four years into withdrawal, Kelly's immune-compromised skin caught a dangerous virus. Hospitalized with a high fever, she didn't know if she would survive.

"That infection changed everything," she recalls. "It burned away my grief and left only the certainty that I had to fight back—even if it cost my life."

It was the moment she stopped being a survivor and became a warrior.

Entering the Arena

In June 2016, while visiting her parents in Michigan, Kelly met ITSAN president Joey Van Dyke for coffee. They talked for hours, and Kelly left with an invitation to join the board. Her first project was a community fundraiser—a small step toward what would become a global advocacy career.

Two years later, she became ITSAN's president. In that role, she launched the *I Wish I Would Have Known* campaign, produced a case-study booklet for clinicians, and co-hosted the landmark Externally Led-Patient Focused Drug Development (EL-PFDD) meeting with the FDA—a six-hour session that elevated TSW into the federal spotlight and secured funding that helped sustain ITSAN for years.

A Healing Embrace

One moment stands apart in her memory. At a National Eczema Association expo, Kelly met a woman from England who dared to ask a prominent dermatologist about TSW during a workshop. The doctor publicly shamed her.

Kelly found her afterward, told her she was proud of her courage, and pulled her into an embrace. They stood together for minutes, Kelly's strength becoming the woman's own. A year later, the woman—a Nigerian—told Kelly that in that moment, all the pain of a lifetime of being talked down to and treated poorly because of her race had culminated in unbearable hurt. Kelly's compassion, she said, was like "a healing balm" to her soul.

"It's like the kindness of God I received during TSW became part of me," Kelly says, "and now I can give it away."

Leading Through Resistance

Kelly's presidency was not without friction. The medical community's indifference was unrelenting, and the internal demands of nonprofit leadership were exhausting. Still recovering at six years into TSW, she pushed through physical setbacks.

Her solution was to build credibility with evidence and connect with decision makers to make them aware of TSW, bringing data and the patient experience to leadership in American Academy of Dermatology, the FDA, Pharmaceutical Industry, Research Community and Dermatology Patient Advocacy Groups. She worked together with Kathy Tullos to develop an international, IRB-approved patient outcomes survey. Published in the *Annals of Allergy and Immunology*, the study has been cited widely and now underpins the push for a dedicated ICD-10 code for TSW.

Allies in the Fight

Even the fiercest fighters need a network—and during her work with ITSAN, Kelly found hers.

There was Dr. Ian Myles of the NIH, whose path first crossed with Kelly's at a National Eczema Association Expo. That chance meeting led to a groundbreaking NIH pilot study on TSW, proving it was not simply atopic dermatitis. The results were published in the *Journal of Investigative Dermatology*, complete with an NIH press release. Myles' introductions also opened doors to the Atopic Dermatitis Research Network, which went on record calling for more TSW research—a turning point for credibility.

There was Tim Smith, a legislative strategist who quietly mentored Kelly and drafted the very language for state and federal resolutions establishing February 3 as TSW Awareness Day. Today, seven states have passed those resolutions, with many more to come.

And there was Dr. Peter Lio—one of the rare US dermatologists, besides Dr. Rapaport, willing to speak publicly and publish about TSW. He co-presented with Kelly at the NEA Expo, addressed the CDC's ICD-10 review board, and worked toward diagnostic criteria—all pro bono.

Kelly is quick to acknowledge the many others: fellow board members past and present, nonprofit leaders, legislative allies, and researchers who each moved the needle in their own way. For Kelly, these collaborations weren't just professional wins—they were proof that in a fight like this, no one wins alone.

The Work Still Ahead

When she looks back, Kelly doesn't measure her presidency by titles or even policy milestones. She measures it in a strong, unified and empowered community, embraces that heal, and the stubborn conviction that TSW's days are numbered.

"I won't stop until I've done my part," she says. "And my part is making sure topical steroids will never again be seen or used the same way."

Passing the Baton

In advocacy, leadership often passes like a baton—one runner exhausted but unwilling to quit, another ready to pick up speed. When Kelly Barta stepped back from ITSAN's presidency in 2019, she placed the torch into the hands of Kathy Tullos—a mother-advocate whose fight for her child's life had already made her a force within ITSAN, and whose tenure would push the movement into new territory.

Kathy Tullos—The Advocate Who Fights for Children

From October 2019 to November 2024, Kathy Tullos led ITSAN with the precision of a nurse, the endurance of a caregiver, and the unshakable focus of a mother who had lived the nightmare firsthand. A Registered Nurse in Pediatrics with a BA in Communications, Kathy had already been part of ITSAN for many years before taking the top role. She joined the board in 2015 and quickly became a cornerstone—creating educational materials, shaping the website, producing brochures and research summaries, and representing ITSAN at medical conferences.

Her presidency marked some of ITSAN's most visible and progressive years, navigating medical resistance, limited resources, and the constant pull of her own son's healing. Her work spanned from launching international research collaborations to presenting directly to the FDA—all while staying deeply connected to the patient community she never stopped serving.

Searching for a Name

Kathy's entry into the TSW world began in July 2013, not for herself but for her four-year-old son. He had been diagnosed with eczema as an infant and prescribed topical steroids—off-label, since the cream wasn't approved for children under two. The results were dramatic at first, but by age three and a half his rashes were worsening, spreading, and shifting from itching to burning. Specialists escalated treatment—stronger potencies, ointments instead of creams, and even occlusion therapy to force absorption—but relief was always short-lived. Soon, the irritation covered nearly his entire body.

As a pediatric nurse, Kathy knew this was no longer "just worsening eczema." Her son had also stopped growing, dropping from the 70th to the 15th percentile for height. An endocrinologist linked the growth delay to head-to-toe topical steroids. A cardiologist discovered a thickened heart wall—another steroid effect—and followed him for five years before finally discharging him in 2018, astonished at his full recovery. These two on-the-record medical opinions gave Kathy the leverage most parents never have: documented justification to stop steroids entirely.

Her Son's Descent

When they stopped treatment, everything got worse—fast. Doctors might have seen this as proof the drugs were needed; Kathy knew better. "Our backs were against the wall," she says. "It wasn't a choice anymore." Her son's withdrawal was brutal: full-body raw skin, hair loss, swollen lymph nodes biopsied to rule out cancer, and the inability to regulate his body temperature. She vacuumed his sheets multiple times a day from the constant shedding. Then came MRSA—an aggressive, hospital-acquired infection that dragged on for 18 months, with antibiotics two weeks out of every month. "When he was on antibiotics, his skin looked better," Kathy says. "It was one of the only times I could exhale."

The Long Climb Back

Fifteen months after stopping steroids, her son's skin was about 80% clear. Kathy secured a home unit for narrow-band UVB phototherapy and treated him three times a week for six months. By the end, his eczema had returned to a manageable baseline—small patches behind the knees or on the ankles, cycling with the seasons. "It pains me to think that by not treating with steroids, he was left with such a minor annoyance—and by treating steroids, we caused so much suffering," she says. "I don't think anyone knows what pure eczema looks like anymore."

A Mother's Anger Becomes a Mission

The turning point wasn't just her son's recovery—it was the medical profession's response. No acknowledgment that steroids had caused the problem. No credit that stopping them had led to healing. Just dismissals: He must have grown out of it. Maybe he was allergic to one ingredient in one cream. As a nurse, she felt the sting of professional judgment. As a mother, she lived under the shadow of Child Protective Services—any specialist could have reported her for noncompliance. "I didn't want other parents to be blamed, suspected, threatened," she says. "It's hard enough to have a sick child." That determination became her compass as ITSAN's president.

Building Bridges to Protect Children

Kathy's leadership centered on one conviction: if the medical community didn't recognize TSW as real, children would remain at risk. Parents can't refuse a doctor's orders without consequences. That meant Kathy had to walk a tightrope—forceful enough to convey the patient experience, measured enough to maintain medical credibility. Her strategy worked. Under her leadership:

- She presented at the Society for Investigative Dermatology in 2022.

- ITSAN launched the "Spark" virtual patient conference in 2021.

- She and Kelly Barta hosted 2 Listening Sessions with the FDA, proposing product label changes and a public health advisory.

- ITSAN partnered with the National Organization for Rare Disorders to develop a patient registry to define TSW's prevalence, natural history, and core symptoms.

- In March 2024, ITSAN's proposal for a dedicated ICD-10 code was accepted for consideration—a step that, if finalized, would revolutionize insurance coverage, disability claims, and diagnostic accuracy.

- Her name is listed as an author representing ITSAN in over 15 scholarly, peer-reviewed articles—achieving more credibility for ITSAN as a patient organization and further legitimizing TSW in the medical and academic world.

A Full Circle Moment

One of her most meaningful milestones came in 2022, presenting alongside Dr. Peter Lio at the NEA Eczema Expo. Years earlier, as a new ITSAN board member, she had nervously approached Lio after a dermatology conference to thank him for his sympathetic work on TSW. "I almost walked past him," she remembers. "But I thought of my son—and the community." Standing beside him years later as a peer presenter was, for her, proof of how far the movement had come. This is the same NEA that refused to let ITSAN attend expos as detailed in Chapter 6.

The Personal Cost

Kathy admits she wanted to quit almost the entire time she was president. "If there had been someone ready to take over, I would have stepped aside in a heartbeat," she says. But no one else stepped forward, so she stayed. The work consumed her days and nights, eroded her boundaries, and often left her with symptoms of PTSD. "What kept me going was simple," she says. "If not me, then who?"

Allies in the Fight

Besides those mentioned assisting in the wins above, there was the expanding circle of board members, volunteers, and patient leaders who made impossible tasks achievable: building the patient registry from scratch, coordinating the Spark conference, and representing TSW at medical meetings where the diagnosis had never before been spoken aloud. "They were the kind of people," Kathy says, "who showed up with their sleeves rolled up, not looking for credit, just determined to get the work done. That's the only way a fight like this moves forward." Kathy said she feels like collaboration is the only option.

Kathy says, "ITSAN was growing so much during that time frame that Kathy recalls she truly couldn't have handled the workload or the emotional toll without her right hand lady Jolene MacDonald." Jolene was a dedicated volunteer for over 2 years, did contract work as well and served on ITSAN's board as secretary, often working 30 hours a week. She answered every email and message with deep care and compassion, updated our supportive doctors lists, created and posted our social media posts, compiled pictures of TSW folks with permissions, wrote our blog, and too much more to list here.

Kathy's decade-plus of service to ITSAN—as board member, executive leader, and president—stands as a record in the organization's history. She left not only structural accomplishments and medical inroads, but an indelible mark of excellence on how ITSAN advocates for its most vulnerable members. **Though no longer president, she continues to direct ITSAN's Patient Registry program, lending her experience and perspective to help move TSW research forward.** Her parting hope: that no parent will ever again have to discover the truth about TSW alone, in an online support group, after years of harm.

When Kathy stepped down as President, she returned the torch to familiar hands—Kelly Barta—whose own scars from TSW and years of board service had prepared her to lead again, this time with even greater reach and determination.

But before Kathy, and Kelly Barta's first term, the organization was led by someone whose calm, steady presence and big heart helped guide ITSAN through important years of growth—and whose own leadership would one day open the door for Kelly Barta's first presidency. That someone was Joey Van Dyke.

Joey Van Dyke—The Steady Hand in the Storm

Taking the helm from the co-founder, from February 2015 to April 2018, Joey Van Dyke picked up the mantle as the second ever president of ITSAN. She served during a period when the organization needed stability more than anything else. She stepped into the role not from a political appointment or corporate boardroom, but from the heart of the TSW community itself—a place she had lived in, suffered through, and worked tirelessly to support. Her leadership would be defined by endurance, personal sacrifice, and a deep, motherly care for the thousands navigating a medical crisis with no official recognition.

Finding ITSAN

Joey first discovered ITSAN the way so many have—by typing desperate search terms into Google late at night. She had been experiencing worsening symptoms without knowing why when she entered the words *"red, burning rash"* into the search bar. The top result was the Addicted Skin website. Joey sent an email, listed her symptoms, and received an immediate, compassionate reply from Kelly Palace. That moment was a lifeline.

She joined the first Google support group—then just twenty people—and quickly became a moderator as the numbers swelled. Soon, she was running point on outreach, advocacy, and resource development, long before she would be called president.

Joey's Descent

Her own battle began in the fall of 2010, when she stopped using topical steroids for a few weeks and erupted in itchy hives across her chest. The triamcinolone she had on hand didn't help. That was the start of a three-year spiral into the darkest, most painful stretch of her life.

The burning and itching were so severe she ended up in the ER twice for nerve pain. She couldn't sleep for more than short stretches, and the constant discomfort led to a dependence on benzodiazepines. Her skin cycled between raw, weeping, and unbearably tight, every movement sending pain signals deep into her nerves.

But even in the middle of her own battle, Joey turned outward—running online groups from her couch, writing letters to universities and news anchors, and carrying ITSAN brochures to every doctor's office she entered. "I never missed a day online from the time I joined that first group until I stepped down as president," she says.

The Turning Point

What transformed Joey from survivor to full-time advocate wasn't just her own suffering—it was watching the syndrome tear through three generations of her family.

Her oldest daughter and granddaughter both went through TSW. Her granddaughter, now fifteen years into the condition, still hasn't fully healed. "I will die on this hill," Joey says, "for the sake of my family and all future generations."

She also saw the endless tide of babies and children entering the support groups—families blindsided by the same preventable harm she had endured. That vision kept her in the fight long after her own skin had healed.

Building a Lifeline

Before becoming president, Joey had already built much of ITSAN's early online infrastructure:

- The first **Red Skin Syndrome** blog, credited with helping future board members identify TSW early.
- A petition for steroid warning labels, signed by Dr. Mototsugu Fukaya himself.
- ITSAN's first private and public Facebook groups, plus a YouTube channel, LinkedIn, Twitter, Instagram, and a monthly newsletter.
- A new forum to handle the growing volume of sufferers.

As president, she managed the website, kept every social media channel active, and answered hundreds of emails from desperate patients. She attended advocacy meetings in Washington, D.C., spoke to dermatologists and medical students, and comforted sufferers in person—from visiting a boy in Seattle going through TSW to sitting in a hospital waiting room with the wife of a man dying from a steroid-related complication.

Leading Through the Storm

When Joey took over ITSAN, it was a difficult time financially and emotionally for the organization. She had no formal training as a nonprofit executive, but she brought two things that couldn't be taught: relentless dedication and an unshakable sense of mission.

She kept the lights on and the work moving with the help of core allies like Susan Ryza and Kathy Tullos, updating the website, running groups, and maintaining the human connections that kept members from falling into despair.

She recalls one night when she stayed on the phone until dawn, talking an ER doctor with TSW through suicidal thoughts—a man who would later become a vocal TSW supporter. "I'll never forget that call," she says. "He told me that if I ever came to California, he would take me to the best restaurant in town."

The Challenges

Externally, Joey faced online trolling from followers of doctors who dismissed TSW, one-star review campaigns, and open ridicule from dermatologists who saw ITSAN as fringe. Internally, the battle was constant: too little funding for research, no budget for staff, and no clear path to an official medical code for the condition.

Her coping mechanism was quiet discipline—deep breathing, prayer, and keeping her private emotions out of public view. "You can't lead well if you're coming from a place of reactivity," she says.

Allies in the Fight

During her presidency, Joey leaned heavily on a small core of dedicated supporters.

Susan Ryza and Kathy Tullos kept ITSAN running during rough patches. Kathy's brother Steve contributed major website updates. "Dr. Fukaya and Dr. Belinda Sheary offered encouragement from across the globe, urging me not to lose hope. Kelly Palace and her husband Mark were always just a phone call away, offering both moral and financial support. They made it possible for me to keep going when I wanted to quit," Joey says. "And I wanted to quit almost every day."

The Steady Hand

By the time she passed the baton to Kelly Barta in 2018, Joey had kept ITSAN alive through some of its most uncertain years. She hadn't just managed an organization—she had held a community together, kept the message alive in the medical space, and made sure no sufferer felt entirely alone.

Her legacy is measured in the thousands of connections she forged, the awareness she raised when few were listening, and the steadiness and big motherly heart she brought to a fight that often felt like chaos.

And before Joey, the torch had been lit for the very first time—by ITSAN's founding president. Kelly Palace built the foundation with Dr. Rapaport and a small circle of committed volunteers—her husband Mark, Joey Van Dyke, Susan Ryza, Kristina Ventura, and others mentioned in the Grassroots Movement chapter—proving that a mighty few can spark a movement that will not be ignored.

Kelly Palace—Patient to President

A Lifetime of Leadership didn't prepare me for the ravages of TSW and watching people suffer. I couldn't talk about the presidents of ITSAN without touching on my own leadership journey. By this chapter, most of my story has already been told—but there are pieces that haven't yet found their place in these pages. Like the women who would follow me, I came to ITSAN through pain, but also with a lifetime of leadership experience that shaped the way I served.

When ITSAN launched, I was no stranger to standing in rooms where I felt alone. Years earlier, I had been the first woman to head coach an NCAA Division I swimming program in the SEC, one of the Power Five conferences—an experience that taught me how to lead under pressure, earn respect, and navigate politics in male-dominated spaces.

A Career Built on Communication

Before that, I had been a journalist and writer, helping produce Pfizer Pharmaceuticals' *Salesforce Magazine* and its companion audio program *Drive Time* for 12,000 members of the company's sales force. I'd written for *Triathlete* magazine, earned All-American honors as a Division I swimmer, captained swim teams, and qualified for the Olympic Trials. These roles demanded grit, communication, and a deep sense of purpose—skills I didn't yet know I would one day pour into leading a global medical movement.

Addicted Skin to ITSAN

You already know the story of my own TSW journey—how I launched *AddictedSkin.org* when no one (except Dr. Marvin Rapaport) was talking about this condition, and how that site became the foundation for ITSAN. By the time I stepped into the role of ITSAN's first president, I had already spent three years in the trenches: fielding desperate emails, moderating online forums, and facilitating teleconferences with Dr. Rapaport that connected sufferers from around the world.

I served as president from ITSAN's official launch in 2012 until 2015—years that blurred into a haze of advocacy, nonprofit building, and daily battles for legitimacy. But I wasn't building bridges between patients and doctors; the doctors wanted nothing to do with us. We were outsiders—branded as outcasts and conspiracy theorists. Outside of our own TSW community, all of whom I mentioned in the early chapters—and our steadfast medical champions, Dr. Rapaport and Dr. Fukaya—those in power didn't just ignore us; they shamed us, ridiculed us, and, at times, openly mocked us.

We were fighting a battle no one wanted to acknowledge, much like another band of determined women more than a century before us—the suffragettes. They were jeered at in the streets, written off in the press, and shut out of the rooms where decisions were made. Yet they refused to yield, laying the groundwork for a future they might never see. In the same way, we four presidents—past and present—worked, and continue to work, so that others can stand on our shoulders and speak the truth without fear.

Memorable Moment

During my presidency, I exchanged hundreds of emails with people around the world suffering from TSW. But I'll never forget the first time I heard one of their voices. Her name was Rochelle. Her email was brief but urgent, and her words carried the unmistakable weight of someone on the edge. I sent her my phone number. Minutes later, my phone rang.

I can still picture the exact spot where I stood when I answered—the world around me seemed to fade as I heard her voice. It was low, shaking, and filled with despair. Rochelle told me she was having thoughts of not wanting to live like this anymore. My heart pounded as I urged her to go to the nearest hospital and speak with a professional. Like so many of us, she did not want to die—but the darkness of TSW can smother hope. Mental health decline is part of the condition.

We talked for a while. She told me that simply hearing my voice, knowing someone else understood, had already made her feel lighter. That moment became a turning point for her. Rochelle went on to become one of ITSAN's fiercest advocates, serving on the board and even allowing her most vulnerable TSW photos to be used in our awareness campaigns.

When I asked Rochelle if I could include this story in the book, she said, "Yes, I will never forget that phone call with you that saved my life. So glad I was able to talk to you that afternoon and find out the real issue... a time when there were no TSW hashtags on social media!"

Stories like this reminded me why the work mattered so much—which made the challenges ahead even harder to face.

Separating From the Good Doctor

One of the most difficult moments of my tenure came in 2013, when Dr. Marvin Rapaport—ITSAN's Co-Founder, someone I adore, and the doctor whose research had saved me—stepped away from the organization. The decision came after differences in vision became too large to bridge: he wanted to focus on direct patient care, especially through telemedicine, while ITSAN needed to remain a patient-led nonprofit capable of lobbying for systemic change. It was heartbreaking, but we believed then, as we do now, that both paths were essential to helping the most people with TSW that we could.

Passing the Baton

By 2015, I stepped away myself—first to care for my mother as she battled Alzheimer's, and then to face my own fight with breast cancer. Stepping down was one of the hardest choices I've ever made. Beyond those obvious pulls on my attention, I was still battling my own skin: massive flares six years after stopping steroids, unrelenting itch, and nights where I averaged two to three hours of fitful sleep for almost a decade. My hands—where I'd used the most potent steroids for the longest—looked and felt like raw hamburger meat. I never left the house without gloves.

I was physically ill and emotionally burned out after so many years of watching such suffering up close. In my opinion, if Joey Van Dyke had not stepped up to lead ITSAN, the organization would have closed its doors. I am forever grateful for her and the amazing leaders who followed.

Lessons in Leadership

My years at the helm of ITSAN taught me that leadership isn't about having all the answers—or staying past your expiration date. I have no doubt that by stepping aside and letting others lead with different talents and skills, ITSAN is in a stronger place today than if I had pushed through the pain and exhaustion I felt. Sometimes, we all need a break.

While I wasn't serving in an official leadership role at ITSAN, I stayed deeply involved—donating regularly, fundraising from the sidelines, and never missing a chance to pass out awareness cards or share TSW's story. That time away also gave me clarity: this movement needed a book like this—to keep the mission alive, to put the truth in print, and to carry hope forward. After years of watching the TSW movement, seeing the entrenched establishment dig in its heels, and filling my journals with those observations, this book finally came into focus.

Four torches. One flame. The hands may change, but the fire still burns brightly—and now, that light is guiding ITSAN into a new era of growth, recognition, and hope.

|||||||||||||||||||||||||||||||||||||||||||||||||||||||||||||||||||||||||||||||||||||||||||||||||||||||||||||||||||||||||||||||||||||||||||||||||||||||||

CHAPTER EIGHTEEN

THE FUTURE

||||||||||||||||||||||||||||||||||||||||||||||||||||||||||||||||||||||||||||||||||||||||||||||||||||||||||||||||||||||||

PICTURE IT.

It's not a hospital ward. It's not a dimly lit pharmacy aisle. It's a city street—alive with color and sound. Balloons bob against the sky, banners ripple in the breeze, and a brass band kicks into a triumphant march. Children with painted faces run ahead of their parents, laughing. Survivors link arms, their skin glowing in the sun. Doctors walk alongside them, not as skeptics but as allies. And up ahead, a banner stretches wide across the street:

WORLD TOPICAL STEROID AWARENESS DAY

Imagine the scene spreading across continents. Tokyo, London, Sydney, Lagos, Los Angeles. Not hidden in Facebook groups, but celebrated in public squares. No longer whispers, but parades. No longer isolation, but community.

For decades, this movement lived in shadows—dismissed as rare, shamed as hysteria, mocked as "phobia." But every year, more people have stepped out of the shadows. A mother raising her voice.

A filmmaker with a camera. A doctor with the courage to say, "I believe you." And like the first follower who joins a lone dancer, their courage transformed ridicule into a movement.

Dr. Rapaport was our lone dancer, swaying on a hilltop of doubt. For decades, he kept the beat alone. Now the crowd is forming—parents, patients, researchers, advocates, and yes, even dermatologists like Dr. Peter Lio. And once the crowd begins to move, history tells us there is no going back.

This is the future. Not a world without topical steroids—they still have a place. But a world where their risks are known, their use is cautious, and every prescription comes with the truth. These drugs can help in the short term, and harm in the long. A world where informed consent isn't optional, but mandatory. Where stewardship replaces silence. Where children are never blindsided by suffering that could have been prevented.

The Tide Is Already Shifting

The future is not some distant dream—it's already unfolding. The tide is turning. More dermatologists are beginning to acknowledge TSW. More research is being done. Patients are no longer hiding, but stepping out of the shadows to share their stories. And with every voice, every study, every doctor who joins, the truth grows louder, harder, and ultimately impossible to silence.

The Definitive Voice on the TSW Problem

In the preface of this book, I told you that no one else could make the claims to write *False Cure*—my family history in medicine, my decade inside Big Pharma, my personal descent into TSW, and my co-founding of ITSAN. But if there is one woman in the world who can speak with equal authority—and perhaps even greater clarity—on how we turn this crisis around, it is **Kelly Barta**, the current president of ITSAN.

And here's the irony: both of us spell our name exactly the same way—**K-E-L-L-Y. The meaning of Kelly is *warrior***. Fitting, because Kelly Barta has proven herself one of the fiercest warriors this movement has ever known. TSW nearly cost her everything: her health, her marriage, even her life. And yet, instead of retreating, she turned her pain into purpose, devoting herself entirely to solving what she calls "the TSW problem."

Barta has carried this fight on her shoulders with unrelenting courage. For me, it is both personal and profound to conclude this book with her words—because if my chapters have traced the arc of this hidden epidemic, her words distill the problem into a single, devastating truth:

> *TSW persists because every link in the health-care chain defers responsibility—approval, education, surveillance, and clinical practice all fall short—so patients are overexposed to topical steroids without informed consent, misdiagnosed when harm appears, and left to fight for recognition while industry incentives push attention toward new drugs instead of fixing the root cause.*

Barta's analysis is blunt: every link in the system has abdicated responsibility. Pre-approval trials were too thin to catch long-term harm. No post-market surveillance ever tracked it. Red flags were buried in journals. Doctors misread withdrawal as "worsening eczema." Universities kept curricula anchored to flawed guidelines. The AAD framed caution as "phobia." The FDA shrugged, calling it a "practice of medicine" issue. Pharma pushed new formulations while burying old harms. NIH and CDC remained largely in the dark, inaccessible and bogged down by competing priorities

The result is structural abdication: patients harmed without consent, misdiagnosed when they worsen, and forced to generate the very evidence the system should have provided. And the greatest risk now, Barta warns, is that history could repeat itself—that new, high-priced drugs could bury the TSW story all over again, swapping one dependency cycle for another, *one false cure for another one,* without ever really looking at the underlying problem, setting patients up for worse outcomes.

Concrete Goals for Tomorrow

The destination is clear:

- **Topical Steroid Awareness Day**—around the world, international and regional recognition that unites patients, families, and physicians in truth and prevention.

- **ICD-10/11 diagnostic codes** dedicated to TSA/TSW—unlocking legitimacy, prevalence, tracking, insurance coverage, and research funding.

- **International Patient Registry** to determine global prevalence and track the TSW patient journey, informing TSW research initiatives.

- **Informed consent as standard practice.** No prescription without a clear conversation: *short-term relief, but long-term risk.*

- **Insurance coverage and disability recognition.** Both short- and long-term disability must be available to patients debilitated by TSW.

- **Medical education reform.** TSW must be part of dermatology, general practice, pediatrics, physician assistant and nursing curricula so future doctors recognize it.

- **Updated clinical guidelines.** AAD and global societies must revise "standard of care" to include TSW, safe-use limits, and tapering protocols.

- **Mandatory post-market surveillance.** Regulators and manufacturers must track long-term safety, not just pre-approval data and take action when necessary.

- **Funded research.** NIH and equivalent agencies must prioritize TSW research grants to determine underpinnings of the condition and viable treatments, along with running natural history studies.

- **Public advisories and warnings.** FDA, Health Canada, TGA, EMA, MHRA, and other governmental regulating bodies must issue clear advisories, label changes, and case reporting requirements.

- **Pharma transparency.** Manufacturers must disclose risks openly, fund safety studies, and stop burying inconvenient data.

- **Stewardship guidelines across specialties.** Dermatology, allergy, respiratory, ophthalmology—must coordinate care and account for cumulative steroid load.

- **Warning labels as stark as tobacco.** Clear, bold, impossible to miss: This product is a corticosteroid with a potency of (X): *May cause addiction and withdrawal.*

- **Funding for safer alternatives** and long-term studies that measure what has been ignored for decades: why some people become dependent and when, and how to treat TSW appropriately so people don't suffer for years.

- **The Marvin J. Rapaport, MD Award of Distinction**—presented annually to the dermatologist who has contributed most to the TSW Movement, with so many worthy candidates that the decision is difficult each year.

- **ITSAN's ultimate goal: to make itself unnecessary.** Because in a just world, no nonprofit should have to exist to expose what medicine itself should have protected against.

Closing Vision

Bad actors will be on the wrong side of history. The profiteers will fade. But the mothers who held burning babies through the night?

The fathers who marched? The doctors who dared? They will be remembered.

One day soon, a child prescribed a steroid cream will also be handed a leaflet that reads: *Short-term use only. Risk of dependency. Monitor closely. This is a steroid.* That child will never know the nightmare you've just read.

And when that day comes, hopefully this book will have been part of the reason why.

Thank you Dr. Marvin J. Rapaport

We started this book with you, and it must end with you as well, because this movement exists only because you refused to look away. You saved countless lives and spared untold suffering. For decades, you stood alone—yet you chose to keep listening, keep documenting, and keep standing for patients when no one else would. You lit a torch in the darkness, and because of you, the world now has a path forward. Our vision for the not-so-distant future is that one day, medicine will honor you, and your contributions to public health will be recognized for what they are—**a legacy worthy of the Nobel Prize in Medicine**.

And we will honor you each year by giving **The Marvin J. Rapaport, MD Award of Distinction**.

As **Thoreau wrote:** *"The man who goes alone can start today; but he who travels with another must wait until that other is ready, and it may be a long time before they get off."* You went alone, and you started. Now, Dr. Rapaport, we hope the world is finally ready to go along with you.

Thank you.

CALL TO ACTION

‖‖‖

✤ **If this book helped you, please leave a review on Amazon.** Did it clarify the evidence? Affirm your experience? Was it well-written, well-researched, and engaging? Your honest reflections guide others.

✤ **If you believe it earns it, a five-star rating will help amplify the message.** Thoughtful five-star reviews from real readers ensure families, clinicians, and journalists can find credible information.

✤ **On contentious topics like this, organized skepticism and denial often flood the ratings with one-star reviews.** Your review helps raise the voice that TSW is real—and keeps deniers from drowning it out.

✤ **Your voice matters—today. Thank you.**

Want to join the fight?

Does your heart call you to advocacy or activism? *We need both.*

At ITSAN's Action Hub, you'll find ways to make an impact—whether by raising awareness, supporting patients, or pushing for policy change. Together we can **PROTECT patients, PROVE the truth, and PREVENT future harm.**

Turn pain into purpose, and purpose into progress. Visit **ITSAN.org** to claim your place in this movement.

Scan the code below for the Action Hub

actionhub.itsan.org

ACKNOWLEDGMENTS

A Community of Courage

To the many who carried the torch before me, beside me, and after me. One of my deepest hopes for this book was to honor the doctors, caregivers, patients, advocates, and activists who have carried this movement forward. Now, as I arrive at the acknowledgments, I find myself almost at a loss for new names to add, because so many have already been woven into these pages.

To Those in the Depths

To those going through topical steroid withdrawal right now: I see you. I know this may feel like the darkest time of your life. The days are long, the nights even longer, and it can seem like there is no way out. Everyone I've known who has endured TSW has gotten better. And often, something unexpected emerges from the suffering: resilience, compassion, and a strength you never asked for but will carry with you forever.

It is my deepest hope that this book has given you validation, helped you realize that this is not your fault, and reminded you that you are part of a global community.

To Dr. Mototsugu Fukaya

In the chapters of this book, I have already honored the research and courage of Dr. Mototsugu Fukaya, but I want to pause here to recognize him more fully and express my gratitude. His partnership has been invaluable to the movement. While Dr. Marvin Rapaport is rightly regarded as the father of the TSW movement, Dr. Fukaya has been one of its most dedicated champions. For decades, he has stood beside patients and advocates, offering not only his scientific expertise but also his steady, compassionate support to ITSAN. Thank you, Dr. Fukaya.

To Jane Jackson Rapaport

With heartfelt appreciation, I acknowledge the many ways you have helped bring this book to life. From gathering research, information, and connections to Dr. Rapaport's work, to hosting a book launch gathering, your steady and generous support and encouragement have been invaluable. Thank you for your commitment, wisdom, and friendship in making this project possible.

To John McGlasson

I owe deep gratitude to John McGlasson—a healed patient of Dr. Rapaport—whose journey from suffering to recovery has become a beacon of hope for so many. Beyond his own healing, John has tirelessly given back to the TSW community by helping Dr. Rapaport manage his Red Skin Syndrome website and producing educational YouTube videos from Dr. Rapaport that spread knowledge, foster good conversation, and provide clarity for patients and families in need. Personally, I am especially thankful to John for serving as a vital coordinator in bringing this book together. Living in close proximity to Dr. Rapaport, John has been an invaluable bridge between us, a trusted friend to Dr. Rapaport, and a thoughtful supporter to me across the country. It was also John's outstanding idea to establish the perpetual annual Marvin J. Rapaport Award of Distinction—a recognition long overdue for those who champion the truth of TSW. Thank you, John. I am so glad you are healed, and that, like me, you were among the fortunate ones to be a patient of this great doctor.

To ITSAN Faithfuls

As the largest and most established organization for the TSW community, ITSAN would not be where it is today without the dedication of the following people—in addition to those already honored in the previous pages:

- **Jodie Ohr** — A TSW warrior prescribed 56 refills of a steroid lotion to use on her face, most likely for a simple make-up reaction. She has been in TSW for nine years and is still fighting. Jodie served on ITSAN's board for six years as either secretary or treasurer, bringing lived experience and steady leadership.
- **Jolene MacDonald** — A mother whose young son went through TSW, Jolene served as ITSAN's secretary and admin assistant for nearly four and a half years. She was, in many ways, the glue that held the organization together during critical years, working tirelessly behind the scenes until life circumstances pulled her away.
- **Natalie Lawton** — The mother of a young adult daughter who endured TSW, Natalie has moderated the ITSAN Facebook group for the past four years and stepped in to manage social media after Jolene left. Few people can handle the constant weight of those groups, but Natalie has been unwavering—a steady, compassionate presence for thousands.
- **Michelle Li** — A TSW survivor herself, Michelle has been working closely with Kathy to develop ITSAN's Patient Registry over the last few years, creating a vital tool for research and recognition.
- **Molly Evans** — Having endured TSW, Molly became ITSAN's first podcast host, lending her voice to amplify stories and raise awareness through a new platform.

- **Janelle Harris** — Another survivor, Janelle stepped up to support ITSAN's fundraising efforts, helping to keep the mission alive and growing.
- **Rochelle Richter** — As a TSW survivor, Rochelle took on the critical role of treasurer, ensuring transparency and trust in the organization's finances. She also allowed her most vulnerable photos during TSW to be used for the cause.
- **Alicia Fasciocco** — Currently navigating TSW herself, Alicia served as ITSAN's secretary before stepping down in 2024 alongside Jodie. Her time in leadership reflected the difficult balance of giving back while still in the depths of the journey.

To Early (Beta) Readers

To my many early readers—family, friends, and even a few strangers—who lent me their eyes, ears, and honesty: your feedback lives in these pages, and I am grateful. Your advice and questions helped refine the clarity, flow, and impact of this book, and sharpened the message I most needed to share.

Stay in Touch

And to every patient, parent, doctor, and advocate who gave their voice, their time, or their story: this book belongs to you.

If this book mattered to you, please leave a 5-star review on Amazon—your voice helps lift the truth above the deniers who will undoubtedly leave 1-star reviews to drown it out.

Thank you! I'd love to hear your feedback in the form of an Amazon review, and you can also reach me at AddictedSkin@gmail.com.

My hope is that by the time you reach this point in the book, it is clear that this fight has spanned decades, and that these countless brave and brilliant people will one day celebrate together when this epidemic is finally recognized—and extinguished.

APPENDIX 1

REBUTTALS FOR SKEPTICS

||||||||||||||||||||||||||||||||||||||||||||||||||||||||||||||||||||||||||||||||||||||||||||||||||||||||||||||||||||||||||

Common objections—
and the evidence that answers them.

Here are the 12 most common objections about TSW—and their **answers from Board Certified Dermatologist, Dr. Marvin Rapaport.**

Every one of these points has already been addressed throughout the chapters of this book, with more detail, but this appendix can be used as a quick-reference guide for patients, advocates, and skeptics. Endnotes below verify all referenced sources.

1. Topical steroid withdrawal isn't even a real condition. I've never seen a single case in my career.

A: You can't diagnose what you don't believe exists. TSW is misdiagnosed every day as "severe eczema" or "a flare," often after stopping steroids—exactly when most clinicians stop watching the patient.[6, 7, 8, 9, 10, 11, 31, 33] Dermatology flagged "steroid addiction" nearly 50 years ago.[12, 36]

2. There's no science behind TSW; it's all anecdotal and crowdsourced. If it were real, we'd have dozens of peer-reviewed studies.

A: We do, in fact, have dozens of peer-reviewed studies. The science spans decades. Foundational clinical papers define corticosteroid addiction/withdrawal, with prevalence data and diagnostic patterns; multiple **systematic reviews** and **prospective cohorts** (including pediatric series) document consistent features; **large international surveys** and a **UK regulator review** further corroborate it.[6, 8, 13, 20, 21, 22, 23, 28, 29, 31, 32, 34] **Over 100 peer-reviewed clinic articles have been published recognizing Red Skin Syndrome, TSA, TSW and TCS damage. That's science.**

3. Withdrawal is just a flare of uncontrolled eczema.

A: Then account for the burning pain, spreading erythema to previously unaffected areas, marked temperature/touch hypersensitivity, edema, and oozing that persist for months to years after cessation—a classic drug-withdrawal pattern documented in case series, surveys, and longitudinal cohorts.[6, 7, 8, 9, 10, 11, 20, 21, 22, 23, 31, 33] And account for why steroids stop working on many people, producing dependency and rebound instead of relief.[5, 36] Eczema itches and is localized; TSW burns and affects body systems beyond the skin.

4. If this were real, the FDA or AAD would have issued warnings by now.

A: Regulators are often the last to move—see asbestos, tobacco, opioids.[5, 12, 49] The FDA leans heavily on post-market reporting, which fails when clinicians don't recognize or report the syndrome, a weakness documented by the Institute of Medicine.[40] Meanwhile, the agency issues safety communications on far less consequential rebound phenomena (e.g., cetirizine "withdrawal itch") while leaving topical steroids without a single boxed warning.[39, 42, 50] This selective silence—contrasted with the scale of published TSW evidence—reveals regulatory alignment with industry, not absence of risk.[43, 44, 45]

5. This is rare. I've prescribed topical corticosteroids for decades, and my patients are fine.

A: Rare compared to what? In Japan, adult TSA prevalence is conservatively estimated at 12% among patients treated for atopic dermatitis.[31] Global AD prevalence is 10-25% worldwide.[31] In the U.K., a leading GP estimated up to 10% of severe eczema cases could actually be TSW.[26] Surveys confirm large numbers of patients reporting steroid-induced harm,[32] and longitudinal cohorts document withdrawal patterns across age groups.[33] For perspective: **multiple sclerosis affects ~0.3% of the population, Crohn's ~0.3-0.5%.** Calling TSW "rare" misrepresents both the math and the lived reality. For an exact breakdown of prevalence see chapter 5. **As many as 120-130 million people worldwide—adults and children combined—may be living with topical steroid addiction or withdrawal.**

6. Your stories are just anecdotes. There's no science.

A: Clinical science begins with patterns in lived cases. When thousands of patients across countries report the same post-steroid trajectory—burning, erythema, hypersensitivity, edema, and oozing—with identical features and timelines, and those match published series, that's a signal, not noise.[6, 7, 8, 9, 10, 11, 28, 29, 31, 33] Surveys and systematic reviews further consolidate these patterns across continents.[13, 32, 34] The consistency across case reports, prospective cohorts, pediatric reviews, and regulator analyses makes clear: this is not anecdote; this is reproducible evidence. **Over 100 peer-reviewed clinic articles have been published recognizing Red Skin Syndrome, TSA, TSW and TCS damage. That's science.**

7. TSW is an internet conspiracy fueled by anti-medicine bloggers.

A: The first warnings predate the internet by decades. Dermatologists themselves documented "steroid addiction" as early as 1979.[36] Since then, multiple peer-reviewed case series, mechanistic studies, prevalence estimates, systematic reviews, pediatric reports, and regulator analyses have reinforced the evidence.[6, 7, 8, 9, 10, 11, 28, 29, 31, 33, 34] Patients didn't invent this; they lived it. The web simply connected those harmed and gave their voices reach.

8. Patients just used their steroids incorrectly.

A: Many followed instructions precisely and still developed dependence—even at so-called "safe" doses.[8, 31, 33] Case series and cohorts document withdrawal in compliant patients using guideline-based regimens.[6, 7, 20, 21, 22, 23] In India, widespread over-the-counter steroid blends and fairness creams created dependence in users who thought they were applying cosmetics, not hormones.[13, 14, 15, 16, 17, 18] The problem is not simply "user error"; it is the addictive pharmacology of topical corticosteroids.

9. The benefits outweigh the risks.

A: Short-term benefit in select cases is not in dispute; what's been underestimated is the **documented, cumulative, multi-route risk** and the absence of informed-consent/monitoring to match it. Comprehensive reviews and mechanistic papers detail **HPA-axis suppression, skin atrophy, ocular complications, osteoporosis, infection risk, metabolic and mood effects** from topical exposure alone.[51, 52, 61] Stewardship pieces and meta-analyses show **systemic absorption across routes** (topical, inhaled, intranasal, ocular), with **additive suppression** when routes are combined.[53, 54, 55, 58] Guidance from endocrine and patient-advocacy bodies now treats **all steroid routes as cumulative**, recommending safety cards and lifetime-exposure minimization.[56, 57] Ophthalmic data confirm that a **tiny eye**

drop can absorb systemically (≤80%) and carry steroid risks.[59, 60] Meanwhile, regulators have repeatedly uncovered **hidden steroids in consumer products** (cosmetic fade creams, lip/face "botanicals," Skin-Cap, Mario Badescu)—exposing unsuspecting users to pharmacologic doses **without any informed consent**, and prompting seizures, suspensions, and suits.[63, 64, 65, 66, 67, 68] Finally, dermatology-focused reviews note **cumulative percutaneous load** over time,[69] while market reports and annual filings underscore powerful financial incentives to **extend steroid use via reformulations and mass consumer channels**—conditions under which risks are most likely to be downplayed rather than proactively mitigated.[70, 71, 72, 73, 74] In that light, "benefits outweigh risks" is true **only** when risks are fully disclosed, routes are counted together, monitoring is real, and safer alternatives/exit plans exist—conditions too often absent in standard practice.[51, 52, 53, 56, 58]

10. Patients with TSW just have steroid phobia.

A: Phobia implies irrational fear—but patients with topical steroid withdrawal are anything but irrational. The vast majority used topical corticosteroids freely and trustingly, often for years, following prescriptions exactly as directed or buying them over-the-counter without hesitation.[8, 31, 33] How can someone who has applied these creams to their infant's face, their own eyelids, or over large body areas be called "phobic"? What they are now is **steroid-informed**: they learned through lived injury that dependence, rebound, and systemic effects are real.[6, 7, 8, 9, 10, 11, 20, 21, 22, 23, 28, 29, 32, 34] Far from hysteria, this knowledge is grounded in clinical papers spanning decades, systematic reviews, pediatric case series, global prevalence data, and even regulator-acknowledged reports. To dismiss patients as "phobic" is not science—it is a rhetorical weapon that erases both their history of compliant use and the mountain of evidence documenting harm.

11. TSA/TSW only happen with long-term use of high-potency steroids.

A: Not true. Dependence and withdrawal have been reported even with mild agents like 1% hydrocortisone and after relatively short courses.[8, 20, 21, 22, 31] Potency matters, but so do site of application, integrity of the skin barrier, frequency, and cumulative duration.[51, 52, 69] Infants and children are particularly vulnerable, as thin skin and occlusion (e.g., under diapers) amplify absorption.[22, 29, 32] Case series, reviews, and surveys show that even so-called "safe" steroids like hydrocortisone can trigger addiction and withdrawal when used under typical prescribing patterns.[6, 7, 23, 33]

12. If topical steroid withdrawal is a real entity, why don't we see it in dermatosis with lupus, lichen sclerosus or cutaneous T cell lymphoma where patients might be on potent topical corticosteroids for years? (For you, @Dr.Deshan on IG)

A: The underlying disease course is critical. Atopic dermatitis is relapsing–remitting, itchy, inflammatory, and often widespread—a pattern that encourages chronic, escalating steroid use across large body surface areas, with frequent step-ups in potency and duration.[7, 8] By contrast, lupus, lichen sclerosus (LS), and cutaneous T-cell lymphoma (CTCL) tend to be more focal or episodic, and are often treated intermittently or with multimodal regimens rather than the "paint the patient" approach common in eczema.[52, 69] In addition, eczema skin has intrinsic barrier defects, such as filaggrin mutations and high transepidermal water loss, which increase percutaneous absorption of corticosteroids.[51] LS lesions and CTCL plaques may allow localized penetration, but the surrounding skin is usually intact, reducing cumulative systemic exposure, while lupus rashes are often photo-induced and intermittent.

Clinical interpretation bias also matters: in eczema, worsening after steroid withdrawal is typically written off as a "flare," while in lupus, LS, or CTCL, physicians attribute disease activity to the auto-immune or neoplastic process. Yet regulators now warn that topical steroid withdrawal can mimic flare and be missed.[34] Moreover, while LS patients may use super-potent agents such as clobetasol, the treatment field is often limited (e.g., genital or perianal skin), keeping total drug exposure far below that of whole-body eczema treatment.[13, 33] Similarly, CTCL therapies rotate between steroids, phototherapy, and systemic drugs, making continuous long-term steroid monotherapy less common.

It's also important to emphasize that TSW is a dependency syndrome, not a universal outcome—just as not every opioid user becomes addicted. Risk rises sharply in scenarios of high-dose, chronic, diffuse application on barrier-impaired skin, which is archetypal for eczema.[8, 31] Pediatric patients are especially vulnerable, with thinner skin, higher surface area-to-body weight ratios, and impaired barrier function, and numerous reports confirm HPA-axis suppression, iatrogenic Cushing's, and growth effects from topical steroid use in children.[51, 52] Taken together, the evidence shows that TSW emerges in the contexts most conducive to dependency: chronic, escalating, whole-body treatment on impaired skin barriers—explaining why it is most frequently recognized in atopic dermatitis and less so in lupus, LS, or CTCL.

References

1. Posit #1 — TSW is real.

2. Posit #2 — Prevalence is far higher than admitted.

3. Posit #3 — The harm is real and preventable.

4. Posit #4 — Patterns match globally.

5. Posit #5 — The medical establishment has ignored warning signs for decades.

6. Rapaport MJ, Rapaport V. *Eyelid dermatitis to red face syndrome to cure: clinical experience in 100 cases. J Am Acad Dermatol.* 1999;41(3 Pt 1):435–442.

7. Rapaport MJ, Rapaport V. *Prolonged erythema after facial laser resurfacing or phenol peel secondary to corticosteroid addiction. Dermatol Surg.* 1999;25(10):781–784.

8. Rapaport MJ, Lebwohl M. *Corticosteroid addiction and withdrawal in the atopic: the red burning skin syndrome. Clin Dermatol.* 2003;21(3):201–214.

9. Rapaport MJ, Rapaport VH. *Serum nitric oxide levels in "red" patients: separating corticosteroid-addicted patients from those with chronic eczema. Arch Dermatol.* 2004;140(8):1013–1014.

10. Rapaport MJ, Rapaport V. *The red skin syndromes: corticosteroid addiction and withdrawal. Expert Rev Dermatol.* 2006;1(4):547–561.

11. Rapaport MJ. *Rebound vasodilation from long-term topical corticosteroid use. Arch Dermatol.* 2007;143(2):268–269.

12. Hanna-Attisha M, LaChance J, Sadler RC, Schnepp AC. *Elevated blood lead levels in children associated with the Flint drinking water crisis: A spatial analysis of risk and public health response. Am J Public Health.* 2016;106(2):283–290.

13. Lindberg I, et al. *Topical steroid withdrawal: A survey of international patients. Dermatitis.* 2021;32(5):301–309.

14. Sheary B, et al. *Topical steroid withdrawal: A primer for GPs. Aust Fam Physician.* 2016;45(8):584–587.

15. Sheary B, et al. *Topical steroid withdrawal: Adult cohort study of 55 patients. Australas J Dermatol.* 2018;59(2):91–97.

16. Sheary B, et al. *Topical steroid withdrawal in children: A case series of 10 patients. Clin Exp Dermatol.* 2019;44(7):787–793.

17. Sheary B, et al. *Topical steroid withdrawal: A two-year pro-spective study of quality of life in adults ceasing long-term use. Dermatitis.* 2021;32(6):406–414.

18. Hajar T, Leshem YA, Hanifin JM, Nedorost ST, Lio PA, Paller AS. *A systematic review of topical corticosteroid withdrawal ("steroid addiction") in patients with atopic dermatitis and other dermatoses. J Am Acad Dermatol.* 2015;72(3):541–549.

19. Juhász MLW, Cohen JM, Mesinkovska NA. *Topical steroid addiction and withdrawal in children: A systematic review. Pediatr Dermatol.* 2017;34(6):593–601.

20. Fukaya M. *Topical steroid addiction in atopic dermatitis. Drug Healthc Patient Saf.* 2014;6:131–138.

21. Silverberg JI, et al. *Patient-reported harm from topical steroids: A multinational survey. J Am Acad Dermatol.* 2024.

22. Sheary B, et al. Longitudinal Australian clinic cohorts on TSW. *Aust Fam Physician* 2016; *Australas J Dermatol* 2018; *Clin Exp Dermatol* 2019; *Dermatitis* 2021.

23. UK Medicines and Healthcare products Regulatory Agency (MHRA). *Topical steroid withdrawal reactions: A review of the evidence.* 2021.

24. Kligman AM, Frosch PJ. *Steroid addiction. Arch Dermatol.* 1979;115(4):459–460.

25. U.S. Food and Drug Administration. Warning Letter re: unapproved foam sunscreens. Aug 6, 2025.

26. U.S. Food and Drug Administration; *The Medical Letter.* "Cetirizine Withdrawal Itching." Drug Safety Communication, May 2025.

27. U.S. Food and Drug Administration. DailyMed drug labels for clobetasol foam (Impeklo), triamcinolone, betamethasone — no boxed warning.

28. Institute of Medicine. *The Future of Drug Safety: Promoting and Protecting the Health of the Public.* Washington, DC: National Academies Press; 2007.

29. U.S. Food and Drug Administration. Drug Safety Communication: Cetirizine withdrawal itch. May 2025.

30. U.S. Food and Drug Administration. *At a Glance: FY 2024.* Oct 2024.

31. U.S. Food and Drug Administration. *FY 2024 PDUFA Financial Report,* Table 11, p. 6.

32. Spherical Insights. *Topical Corticosteroids Market Report,* 2022; DataIntelo. *Topical Steroids Market Forecast,* 2023.

33. U.S. Food and Drug Administration. NDA Approval, OLUX Foam (clobetasol propionate), 2000; Connetics SEC Filing, OLUX-E, 2007.

34. *New York Times.* "2 Paths of Bayer Drug in 80's: Riskier Type Went Overseas." May 22, 2003. *The Guardian.* "Bayer Sold HIV-Contaminated Blood Products." May 23, 2003.

35. U.S. Food and Drug Administration. *Boxed Warnings Overview.* 2024.

36. Hengge UR, Ruzicka T, Schwartz RA, Cork MJ. *Adverse effects of topical glucocorticosteroids. J Am Acad Dermatol.* 2006;54(1):1–15.

37. Dhar S, Seth J, Parikh D. *Systemic Side-Effects of Topical Corticosteroids. Indian J Dermatol.* 2014;59(5):460–465.

38. DiRuggiero D, DiRuggiero M. *The Systemic Impact of Topical Corticosteroids in Dermatology. J Clin Aesthet Dermatol.* 2025;18(1–2 Suppl 1):S16–S20.

39. Allen DB. *Systemic effects of intranasal steroids: an endocrinologist's perspective. J Allergy Clin Immunol.* 2000;106(4):S179–S190.

40. Sowerby LJ, Fowler J. *Systemic absorption of intranasal corticosteroids may have systemic effects and can add to overall corticosteroid load. CMAJ.* 2014;186(16):1241–1245.

41. Society for Endocrinology (UK). *Exogenous steroids in adults – adrenal insufficiency guidance.* 2021.

42. Global Allergy & Asthma Patient Platform (GAAPP). *Steroid Stewardship Initiative.* 2023.

43. Besemer F, et al. *Adrenal insufficiency in corticosteroid use: a systematic review. Lancet Diabetes Endocrinol.* 2021;9(12):863–872.

44. Medsafe NZ. *A drop in the eye has widespread ripples. Prescriber Update.* Dec 2019.

45. Farkouh A, et al. *Systemic side effects of eye drops: a pharmacokinetic perspective. Clin Ophthalmol.* 2016;10:2433–2441.

46. Schäcke H, Döcke WD, Asadullah K. *Mechanisms involved in the side effects of glucocorticoids. Pharmacol Ther.* 2002;96(1):23–43.

47. National Eye Institute. *Corticosteroids and Eye Health.* Fact Sheet, 2022.

48. Campbell J, Perez M, Woolery-Lloyd H. *Hidden Topical Corticosteroids in Cosmetic Fade Creams Sold in the U.S. J Drugs Dermatol.* 2024;23(6).

49. *Restaino v. Mario Badescu Skin Care, Inc.* Class Action Complaint. 2013.

50. Korean Ministry of Food and Drug Safety. Suspension of Mario Badescu creams containing undisclosed steroids. Regulatory Notice, 2013.

51. *Cheminova America Corp. v. Corker,* 726 So. 2d 1237 (Ala. 1999). (Skin-Cap/undisclosed clobetasol.)

52. U.S. Food and Drug Administration. *Warning: Skin-Cap aerosol spray may contain undisclosed corticosteroids.* Advisory, Oct 2024.

53. Health Canada. *Summary of Enforcement Notifications: Cosmetic and Skin-Lightening Products.* 2022.

54. Hengge UR, Ruzicka T, et al. *Topical glucocorticoids and systemic side effects. Curr Opin Investig Drugs.* 2000;1(3):301–309.

55. GSK plc. *Annual Report 2024.* (Trelegy Ellipta net sales $3.46B).

56. AstraZeneca plc. *Annual Report 2024.* (Symbicort ~$2.9B; Breztri ~$978M).

57. Market Research Future. *Global Corticosteroids Market Report 2024.* (~$5.2B; CAGR 7.5%).

58. GlobalData Healthcare. *Topical Corticosteroids Market Analysis.* 2024. (~$8.4B global).

59. Haleon plc. *Annual Report 2024.* (Consumer Health revenue £11.2B; Respiratory Health 15% incl. Flonase).

60. Farkouh A, et al. *Systemic side effects of eye drops: a pharmacokinetic perspective. Clin Ophthalmol.* 2016;10:2433–2441.

61. Schäcke H, Döcke WD, Asadullah K. *Mechanisms involved in the side effects of glucocorticoids. Pharmacol Ther.* 2002;96(1):23–43.

62. National Eye Institute. *Corticosteroids and Eye Health.* Fact Sheet, 2022.

63. Campbell J, Perez M, Woolery-Lloyd H. *Hidden Topical Corticosteroids in Cosmetic Fade Creams Sold in the U.S. J Drugs Dermatol.* 2024;23(6).

64. *Restaino v. Mario Badescu Skin Care, Inc.* Class Action Complaint. 2013.

APPENDIX 1: REBUTTALS FOR SKEPTICS

65. Korean Ministry of Food and Drug Safety. Suspension of Mario Badescu creams containing undisclosed steroids. Regulatory Notice, 2013.

66. *Cheminova America Corp. v. Corker*, 726 So. 2d 1237 (Ala. 1999). (Skin-Cap/undisclosed clobetasol.)

67. U.S. Food and Drug Administration. *Warning: Skin-Cap aerosol spray may contain undisclosed corticosteroids.* Advisory, Oct 2024.

68. Health Canada. *Summary of Enforcement Notifications: Cosmetic and Skin-Lightening Products.* 2022.

69. Hengge UR, Ruzicka T, et al. *Topical glucocorticoids and systemic side effects. Curr Opin Investig Drugs.* 2000;1(3):301–309.

70. GSK plc. *Annual Report 2024.* (Trelegy Ellipta net sales $3.46B).

71. AstraZeneca plc. *Annual Report 2024.* (Symbicort ~$2.9B; Breztri ~$978M).

72. Market Research Future. *Global Corticosteroids Market Report 2024.* (~$5.2B; CAGR 7.5%).

73. GlobalData Healthcare. *Topical Corticosteroids Market Analysis.* 2024. (~$8.4B global).

74. Haleon plc. *Annual Report 2024.* (Consumer Health revenue £11.2B; Respiratory Health 15% incl. Flonase).

APPENDIX 2

DR. RAPAPORT'S KEY FINDINGS

This appendix preserves a selection of the critical observations of Dr. Marvin J. Rapaport, widely regarded as the leading expert on topical steroid addiction and withdrawal. Across more than four decades, Dr. Rapaport has compiled an extensive record of clinical experience, research, and analysis that documents both the harms of long-term steroid use and the reality of withdrawal. **Patients continue to come to his Los Angeles office from all over the world. He has helped to heal countless patients over the decades he has studied and treated this condition.** On my own visits while healing from TSW, I would often encounter others who had traveled great distances seeking his care; I particularly remember meeting a woman from Sweden who was in such severe pain that she could not sit down for nearly six months.

What is presented here is not the full corpus of his work, but a curated set of his most valued charts and graphs—materials he considered central to understanding the scope and significance of this condition. Together, they form a historical record of his persistence and findings, offering future clinicians, researchers, and patients a foundation upon which to build.

The two-page flowchart found in this appendix illustrates the typical progression Dr. Rapaport has documented in patients developing topical steroid addiction (TSA) and withdrawal (TSW). It traces how patients move from initial use to dependency, and eventually into the cycle of worsening symptoms that steroids themselves perpetuate. To frame this visual, here is a note from Dr. Rapaport: "TSW occurs all during TSA. When patients stop steroids, withdrawal quickly appears, only to be covered up again by renewed steroid use, topically or systemically. In reality, TSW is often being experienced after just two to six weeks of steroid usage—it is merely suppressed for a moment."

The references from which the information in this appendix is drawn can be found after the final table.

List of Charts and Tables in Appendix 2

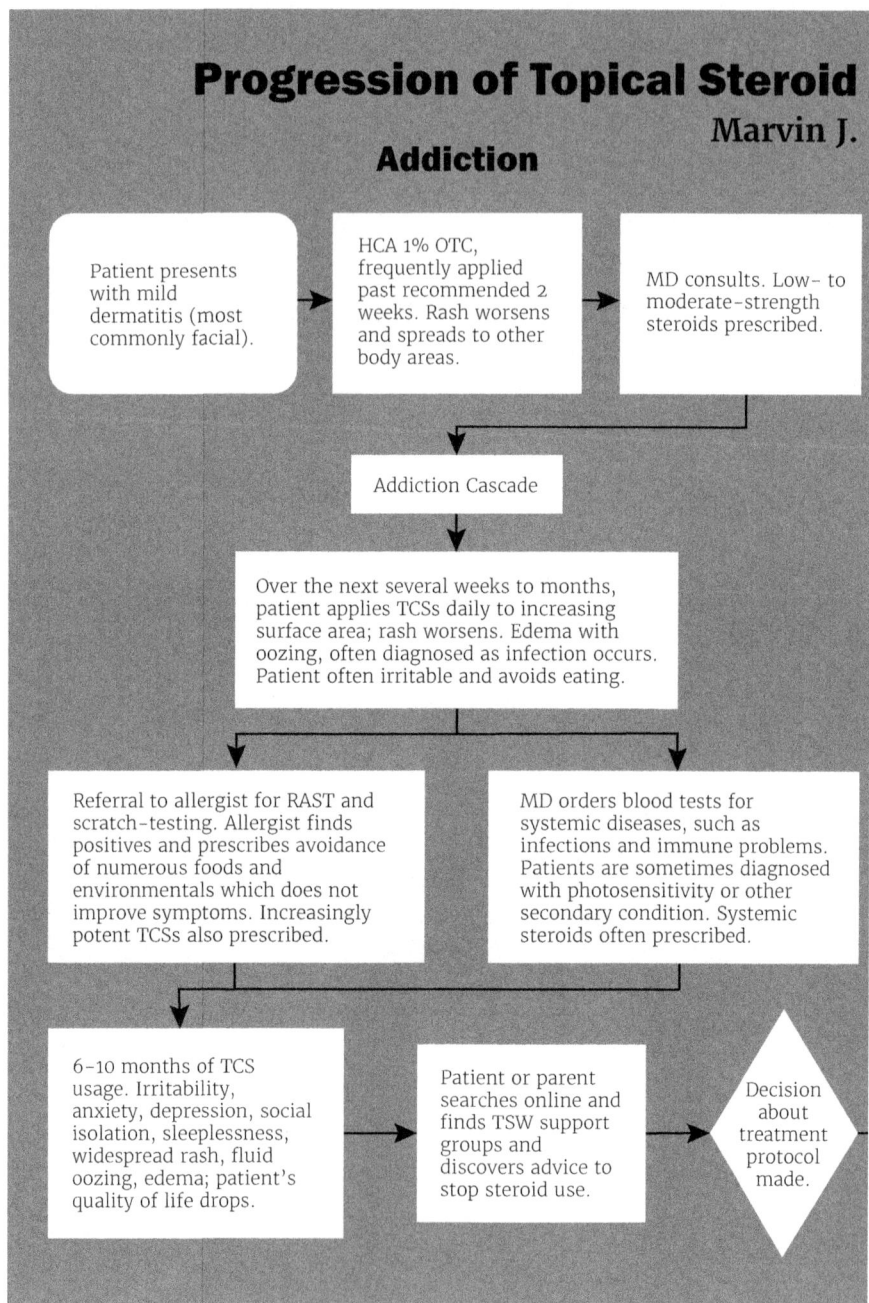

Progression of Topical Steroid Addiction

Marvin J.

Patient presents with mild dermatitis (most commonly facial).	HCA 1% OTC, frequently applied past recommended 2 weeks. Rash worsens and spreads to other body areas.	MD consults. Low- to moderate-strength steroids prescribed.

Addiction Cascade

Over the next several weeks to months, patient applies TCSs daily to increasing surface area; rash worsens. Edema with oozing, often diagnosed as infection occurs. Patient often irritable and avoids eating.

Referral to allergist for RAST and scratch-testing. Allergist finds positives and prescribes avoidance of numerous foods and environmentals which does not improve symptoms. Increasingly potent TCSs also prescribed.

MD orders blood tests for systemic diseases, such as infections and immune problems. Patients are sometimes diagnosed with photosensitivity or other secondary condition. Systemic steroids often prescribed.

6-10 months of TCS usage. Irritability, anxiety, depression, social isolation, sleeplessness, widespread rash, fluid oozing, edema; patient's quality of life drops.

Patient or parent searches online and finds TSW support groups and discovers advice to stop steroid use.

Decision about treatment protocol made.

(TCS) Addiction and Withdrawal
Rapaport, MD

Withdrawal

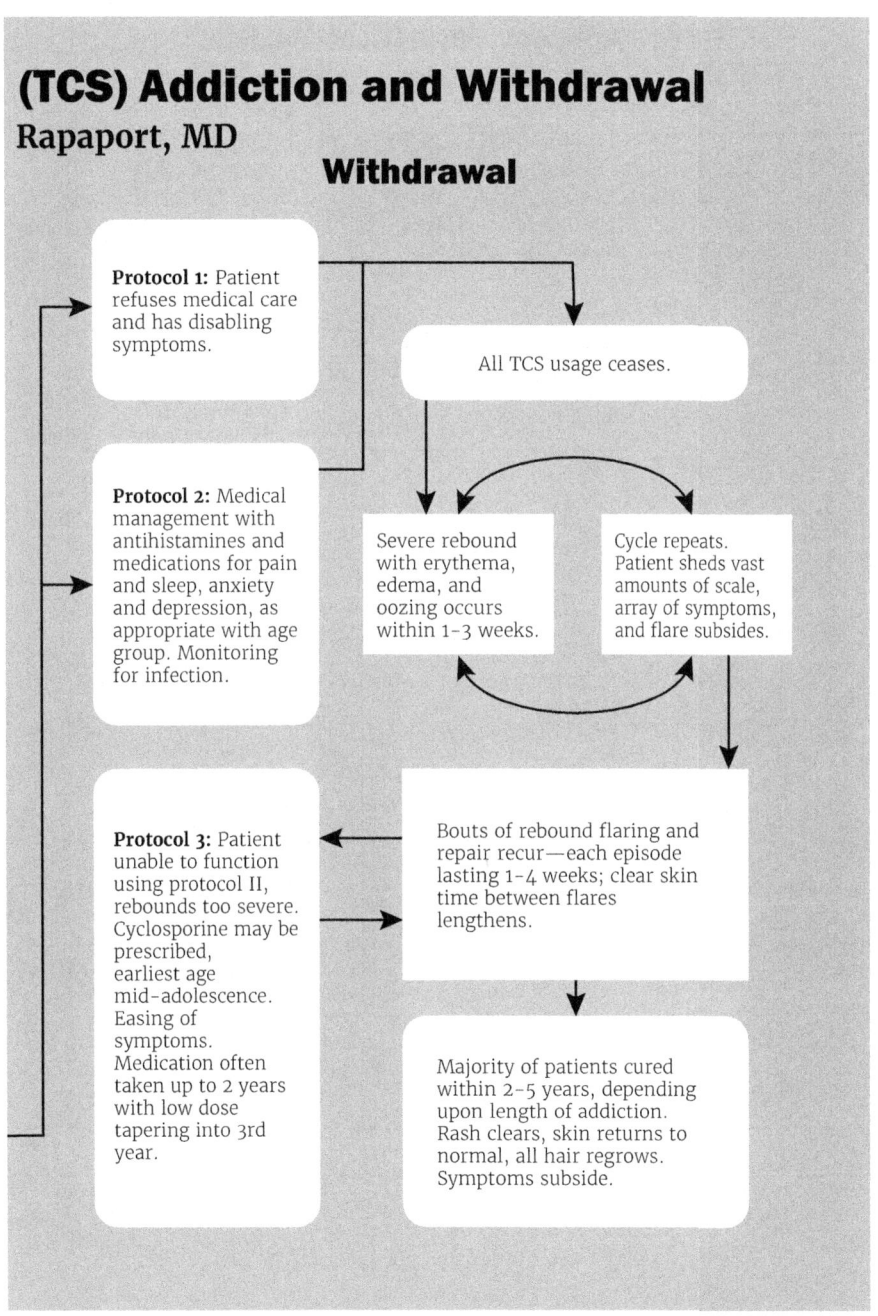

Protocol 1: Patient refuses medical care and has disabling symptoms.

All TCS usage ceases.

Protocol 2: Medical management with antihistamines and medications for pain and sleep, anxiety and depression, as appropriate with age group. Monitoring for infection.

Severe rebound with erythema, edema, and oozing occurs within 1–3 weeks.

Cycle repeats. Patient sheds vast amounts of scale, array of symptoms, and flare subsides.

Protocol 3: Patient unable to function using protocol II, rebounds too severe. Cyclosporine may be prescribed, earliest age mid-adolescence. Easing of symptoms. Medication often taken up to 2 years with low dose tapering into 3rd year.

Bouts of rebound flaring and repair recur—each episode lasting 1–4 weeks; clear skin time between flares lengthens.

Majority of patients cured within 2–5 years, depending upon length of addiction. Rash clears, skin returns to normal, all hair regrows. Symptoms subside.

Table 1a. Atopic Dermatitis: Varying Patterns from the 1800s to the Present

Patterns of Disease		1800s–1980s	1980s–Present
Overall Pattern		Hanifin and Rajka's 1980 criteria cite typical onset at 2–6 months; onset after 5 years of age is virtually nonexistent. Maintained by AAD until recently.	Onset at any time. "Adult-onset" is a distinct phenotype.
Clinical Presentation	**Under 18 Months**	Erythematous and edematous papules, largely on the face. Diaper area spared.	Generalized erythematous, oozing rash, often involving diaper area.
	Childhood	*Localized*, lichenous lesions especially in flexural folds, sides of neck, wrists, and/or ankles. Pruritus caused by skin irritation, such as from wool clothes.	Worsening total body erythroderma with edema and oozing. Increasing usage and strength of steroids, topically and systemically.
	Adulthood	Incidence in adulthood is very rare and not discussed in the literature. 90% or more of patients experience "burn out" before puberty. Possibility of minor relapse in adolescence.	Inability to function; absence from work/school, worsening depression and suicidal ideation. Average age of patients in most recent eczema drug studies is generally between 35–45 years. No patients are described in the literature as cured.
Pathology		Localized lichenification of the epidermis with excoriations.	Generalized spongiosis with erythroderma.
Epidemiology		Prevalence is estimated at 3% of infants and 2–20% of children.	Estimates of 15–20% prevalence among children.
		Thorough literature review did not reveal a significant number of adult cases.	Epidemiologists theorize that AD is a "bimodal" disease with a "second peak" of prevalence mid-life.

Table 1b. Atopic Dermatitis: Causes and Treatments

		1800–1980s	1980s–Present
S&S	**Pruritus**	Moderate.	Severe.
	Burning	Not described in literature.	Very severe in almost all patients.
	Skin Appearance	Dry skin with areas of lichenification.	Severe erythroderma and lichen simplex chronicus.
	Bathing	No intolerance.	Causes severe burning sensation and is invariably avoided.
	Lotions/ Creams	No intolerance.	As above.
	Sun Exposure	Usually curative.	Not tolerated.
	Heat Exposure	Mild pruritus.	Not tolerated.
	Low Humidity	Mild pruritus.	Tolerated.
	Ice Pack Use	Never mentioned in the literature.	Used extensively to ease burning.
	Hair	No alopecia areata.	a) Androgenic alopecia— women only. b) Loss of eyebrows, which regrow.
Causal Factors		Genetic tendency to skin irritation, itchiness and vasoconstriction. Colonization with *Staphylococci* that produce skin irritants and histamine response.	Causes cited include: water hardness, formula feeding, vitamin deficiencies, food and cosmetic allergens, air pollution, household hygiene products.
		Patch testing invariably showed only false positives and even those were rare. Therapeutic avoidance rarely helps ameliorate symptoms.	Atopics should avoid causes cited above in order to avoid "atopic march."

(continued on following page)

Table 1b (*cont.*)

		1800–1980s	1980s–Present
Therapy	Topical	UV light and sun exposure ameliorates rash. Lubricating creams lessen dryness.	Unaffected or worsened by sun exposure when erythrodermic. Creams cause severe burning sensation.
		Weak TCSs used sparingly from 1952–1980s; gave moderate symptom relief. Rebound events not mentioned in the literature.	Increasingly potent TCSs, nothing else relieves symptoms; use of tacrolimus, crisaborole, ruxolitinib.
	Systemic	Antihistamines; prednisone.	The following invariably used in combination with TCSs: a) prednisone b) triamcinolone IM c) methotrexate d) azathioprine e) mycophenolic acid f) cyclosporin.

Table 2. Dermatologic Diseases Treated with Chronic Topical Steroids

	Underlying Disease	Time to Induce Addiction	Characteristics
1.	Atopic Dermatitis	4–8 weeks	See Tables 1a and 1b.
2.	Psoriasis*	1–4 years	Long-term TCS ineffective; flaring and worsening erythroderma now treated with systemic corticosteroids, which subsequently results in exfoliative erythroderma and pustular psoriasis.
3.	Seborrheic Dermatitis*	1–2 years	Severe erythroderma on the face and scalp accompanied by severe burning sensation misdiagnosed as rosacea, photodermatitis, or autoimmune disease.
4.	Asteatosis (Winter Itch)*	3–5 months	Usually affects legs and back, mild erythema and marked spreading and worsening pruritis and burning.

(continued on following page)

Table 2 (*cont.*)

Underlying Disease		Time to Induce Addiction	Characteristics
5.	Post-Laser/ Phenol Peel*	2-4 weeks	Post-op steroids prescribed to lessen erythema, but in fact exaggerate redness, leading to severe burning.
6.	Red Scrotum Syndrome*	2-4 weeks	Mild irritant dermatitis, candidiasis, or tinea, often treated with increasing steroid strengths; patient develops severe burning often with erythema on inner thighs.
7.	Pruritus Vulvae/ Vulvodynia*	2-4 weeks	Initial diagnosis of pruritis treated with steroids results in complaints of stronger pruritis and burning; minimal findings on examination leads to misdiagnosis of neurosis.
8.	Pruritus Ani*	2-10 months	Prolonged scratching and often presence of hemorrhoids.
9.	Contact Dermatitis*	2-10 months	Overtreatment after orthopedic cast on a traumatic wound.
10.	Jock Itch*	2-10 months	Increasing steroid strengths used after initial OTC creams evolved into Red Scrotum Syndrome.
11.	Grover's Disease*	2-10 months	Pruritic papules usually during the summer.
12.	Photo and Contact Dermatitis*	2-10 months	Allergen to be discovered.
13.	Status Cosmeticus*	2-10 months	Intermingling and overtreatment with cosmetic creams and often camouflaged steroids.
14.	Chronic Actinic Dermatitis*	2-10 months	Probable misdiagnosis but appears in literature.
15.	Neurogenic rosacea*	2-10 months	Same as above.
16.	Cheilitis*	2-10 months	Invariably related to sleep apnea and mouth-breathing causing drying of mucosa of lower lip.

These diagnoses exhibited the same skin reactions, namely TSA, RSS, and TSW symptoms, following cessation of TCS use.

||||||||||||||||||||||||||||||||||||||||||||||||||||||||||||||||||||||||||||||||||||||||||||||||||||||||||||||||||||||||||||||||||

References

1. Rapaport MJ, Rapaport V. *Eyelid dermatitis to red face syndrome to cure: clinical experience in 100 cases. J Am Acad Dermatol.* 1999;41(3 Pt 1):435–442.

2. Rapaport MJ, Rapaport V. *Prolonged erythema after facial laser resurfacing or phenol peel secondary to corticosteroid addiction. Dermatol Surg.* 1999;25(10):781–784.

3. Rapaport MJ, Lebwohl M. *Corticosteroid addiction and withdrawal in the atopic: the red burning skin syndrome. Clin Dermatol.* 2003;21(3):201–214.

4. Rapaport MJ, Rapaport VH. *Serum nitric oxide levels in "red" patients: separating corticosteroid-addicted patients from those with chronic eczema. Arch Dermatol.* 2004;140(8):1013–1014.

5. Rapaport MJ, Rapaport V. *The red skin syndromes: corticosteroid addiction and withdrawal. Expert Rev Dermatol.* 2006;1(4):547–561.

6. Rapaport MJ. *Rebound vasodilation from long-term topical corticosteroid use. Arch Dermatol.* 2007;143(2):268–269.

7. Lindberg I, et al. *Topical steroid withdrawal: A survey of international patients. Dermatitis.* 2021;32(5):301–309.

8. Hajar T, Leshem YA, Hanifin JM, Nedorost ST, Lio PA, Paller AS. *A systematic review of topical corticosteroid withdrawal ("steroid addiction") in patients with atopic dermatitis and other dermatoses. J Am Acad Dermatol.* 2015;72(3):541–549.

9. Fukaya M. *Topical steroid addiction in atopic dermatitis. Drug Healthc Patient Saf.* 2014;6:131–138.

APPENDIX 2: DR. RAPAPORT'S KEY FINDINGS

10. Kligman AM, Frosch PJ. *Steroid addiction. Arch Dermatol.* 1979;115(4):459–460.

11. DiRuggiero D, DiRuggiero M. *The Systemic Impact of Topical Corticosteroids in Dermatology. J Clin Aesthet Dermatol.* 2025;18(1–2 Suppl 1):S16–S20.

Printed in Dunstable, United Kingdom

68876124R00167